# Contents

# Preface

There are around 6,000 different kinds of genetic disorders. Many are rare while others are more common, but taken together they are prevalent. It is estimated that one in 25 children is affected by a genetic disorder with 30,000 babies and children newly diagnosed in the UK each year. Some genetic disorders are apparent at birth while others are diagnosed at different stages throughout life. What is important to appreciate is that not all mutations or genetic diseases result in deformities so severe they are incompatible with life. Though we all share 99.9 per cent of our DNA, we are also all genetically unique; we all carry mutations. Our genetic differences influence our physical, mental and behavioural characteristics, together with our health - they make us individual. Crucially, mutations are the driving force of evolution – as our environment constantly changes, so are we constantly evolving to adapt.

In the past, ignorance of genetic abnormalities meant that those afflicted were often ostracised and even feared. Genetic abnormalities may have led to legends of vampires and witches. This book explores the origins and impact of genetic disorders through the lives of celebrities and historical figures who have been afflicted by them. The tales that emerge, tales that are meant to be shared in conversation, are sometimes tragic, but surprisingly often are heart-warming and inspiring.

The book starts with some necessary scientific background in order to allow the reader to fully appreciate what follows. Terminology is inevitable and a glossary has been provided for reference.

# WHAT IS A CELL ?

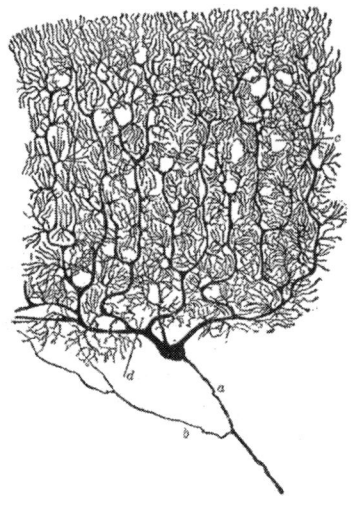

*Although there is no universal agreement as to a definition of life, its biological manifestations are generally considered to be organization, metabolism, growth, irritability, adaptation, and reproduction.*

The Columbia Encyclopaedia, First Edition, first sentence of the article on "life", 1935

A cell is the smallest structure capable of basic life processes, such as absorbing nutrients, expelling waste, and reproducing. Examining a thin section of cork through a homemade microscope Robert Hooke, in 1665, became the first person to see a cell. The first thing that struck him was how the rows of tiny boxes making up the dead wood's tissue looked like the rows of rooms occupied by monks in a monastery, known as cells; hence the name.

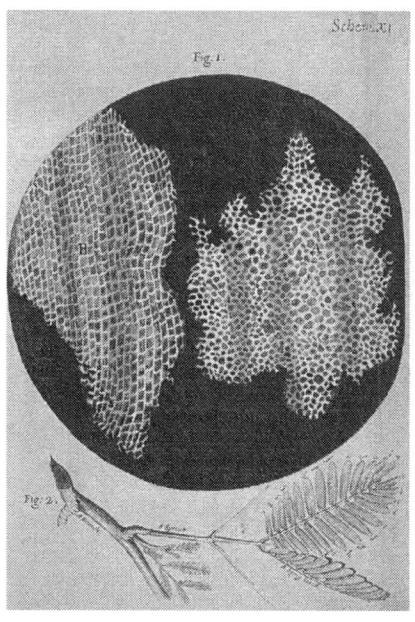

Microscopic view of cells in a sliver of cork. Robert Hooke, 1665

Some microscopic organisms, such as bacteria, exist as a single cell while multicellular organisms, such as ourselves, consist of many different varieties of cells working in concert. We are composed of 20-30 trillion cells. One of the largest human cells is the female egg cell, which is about one millimetre in diameter, while one of the smallest is the male sperm. Cells also vary in shape. They can be round, thin, flat, polygonal, long or branching. Among the longest cells are the nerve cells connecting the end of our toes to the spinal cord spanning half the human body. One of the longest cells in the animal kingdom are the nerve cells running down a giraffe's neck which can be as long as 3 meters.

Cells that make up multicellular organisms are called eukaryotic (Gr. *Eu*; true, *Karyon*; nut, referring to a nucleus) cells and have a nucleus containing DNA. This is in contrast to the simpler prokaryotic cells (Gr, *pro*; before), found only in bacteria, where the DNA mingles freely inside the cell. In addition to the nucleus, eukaryotic cells also contain other organelles including the endoplasmic reticulum, where proteins and lipids (fats) are produced, and the Golgi apparatus where the proteins and lipids are sorted and transported to different places within the cell or body.

Plant and animal eukaryotic cells also contain mitochondria important for the production of energy for the cell. Plants in addition also contain chloroplasts for the same purpose. It is generally accepted that eukaryotic cells evolved from the more primitive prokaryotic cells around 2 billion years ago when bacteria became engulfed and maintained

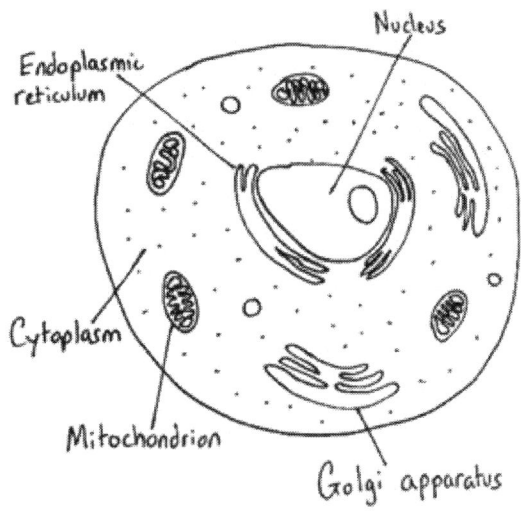

Diagram of a cell

inside other cells for their ability to produce energy thus forming mitochondria and chloroplasts. This idea of once free-living cells living symbiotically inside our cells was used by George Lucus when he wrote the scripts for the *Star Wars* movies – the name he devised, midi-chlorians, is a derivative of mitochondria and chloroplasts. "*Midi-chlorians are a microscopic life form that resides within all living cells*" *Qui-Gon Jinn* said to *Anakin Skywalker*, who had a midi-chlorian count of 20,000. "*Without the midi-chlorians, life could not exist, and we would have no knowledge of the Force. They continually speak to you, telling you the will of the Force*". Jedi warriors were said to have unusually high numbers of these midi-cholirans and they had to train to listen these symbiotes, to allowed them to use the 'Force'. Our muscle cells generally contain around 2,000 mitochondria each. In the same way as Jedi, our mitochondria, in a way, listen to our bodies as they can replicate to increase numbers in our cells following physical exercise for example, allowing our body to produce more energy. Without mitochondria, eukaryotic cell life would not exist. This is evident if we consider the well-known poison, potassium cyanide. This inhibits the ability of mitochondria to produce energy for our cells – 200mg, similar to a pinch of salt, is enough to kill us within minutes.

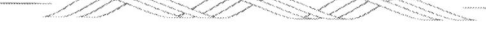

# WHAT IS DNA?

*Knowing what your parents have gives you hints of things, but your genome is a totally unique combination of and interchange of DNA from your parents. There is no one else like you genetically.*

Craig Venter: led the first draft sequence of the human genome

DNA is the hereditary material in all living organisms and is found in every single living cell. In eukaryotic cells, DNA is packaged into structures called chromosomes, which were first observed using a special dye, hence the name (Gr. *chroma*, colour; *soma*, body). An abbreviation of d̲eoxynuclei̲c a̲cid, DNA is a very long molecule made up of a variable sequence of four chemical nucleotides composed of four bases: adenine (A), guanine (G), cytosine (C), and thymine (T). These pair up with each other (A with T and C with G) to form units called base-pairs, which together are arranged in two long strands forming a spiral called a double helix. DNA can replicate as each strand of DNA in the double helix can serve as a template for duplicating the sequence of bases. Therefore, when cells divide each new cell has an exact copy of the DNA.

Human cells contain around 3 billion of the four different bases forming DNA. These are arranged in a specific, yet unique, order to each of us. The bacterial cells *E. coli* contain 4,6 million base pairs, the fruit fly has 160 million base pairs and the dog 2.4

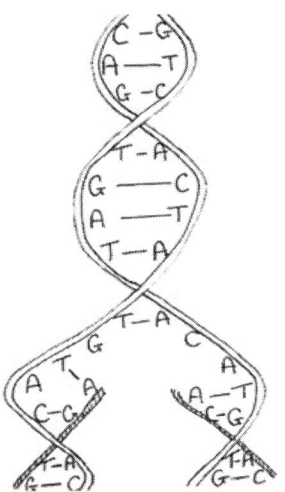

DNA replication

billion. However, the size of the genome often bears little relation to the complexity of the organism; cells of the onion contain five times as much DNA as a human cell!

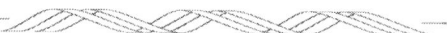

# WHAT IS A GENE?

*If you watch animals objectively for any length of time, you're driven to the conclusion that their main aim in life is to pass on their genes to the next generation.*

David Attenborough

The word "gene" was first used by the Danish botanist Wilhelm Johannsen in 1909 to refer to *"determiners which are present [in the gametes] … [by which] many characteristics of the organism are specified"*, long before DNA was understood. Francis Crick, following his work on the DNA helix and RNA, was then able to define a gene as a stretch of DNA that encodes a piece of RNA that encodes a chain of a protein. He called this the Central Dogma. However, many genes do not code for proteins and produce RNA that has other functions. Hence, a more current definition of a gene is a stretch of DNA that has the potential to create a

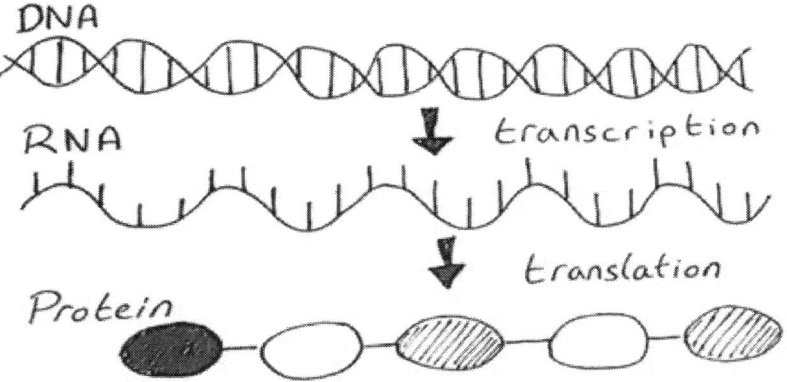

The central dogma: DNA is transcribed into RNA that is translated in protein

characteristic and contribute some function to the organism.

Our DNA contains an estimated 22,000 genes. While sharing over 99.9 per cent identical gene sequences among ourselves as a species, we also share about 96 per cent of our genes with chimpanzees, 80 per cent with mice, 75 per cent with dogs, 50 per cent with the fruit fly (Drosophila) and 30 per cent with yeast. why do many organisms, seemingly less "advanced" than ourselves, have as many genes as we do? One explanation is that many genes are capable of making more than one protein, thus allowing human cells to make the around 80,000-100,000 proteins from our genes that our bodies require.

From Sequencing of the human genome it is estimated that humans have between 20,000 and 25,000 genes. Every person has two copies of each gene, one inherited from each parent. Most genes are the same in all people, but a small number of genes (less than 1 per cent of the total) are slightly different between people. Alleles are forms of the same gene with small differences in their sequence of DNA bases. These small differences contribute to each person's unique physical features. Incredibly, while we do not have the highest amount of DNA in the animal kingdom, we also do not even have the highest numbers of genes. The tiny water flea *Daphnia* has some 31,000 genes.

Genes are given unique names to identify them. Often this relates to the function or significance of the gene. For example, a gene associated with cystic fibrosis is called the cystic fibrosis transmembrane conductance regulator, generally abbreviated to CFTR. Some researchers have displayed a quirky sense of humour when "choosing" a name for a newly discovered gene. Sonic hedgehog is perhaps one of the more famous, describing the human equivalent of a fruit fly gene. The fruit fly gene was named hedgehog because, when mutated, it resulted in fruit fly embryos being covered with hair like a hedgehog. So, when the American scientist, Bob Riddle, discovered the human equivalent of this developmentally important gene, he decided to call it sonic hedgehog after the computer game he enjoyed playing. But there are boundaries to naming a new gene. One research group in 2005 named a gene they had found involved in cancer, after another Japanese video game *Pokémon*, claiming it was an acronym for POK (a previously named family of genes) erythroid myeloid ontogenic. This attracted tongue-in-cheek headlines as "*Pokémon causes cancer*" leading the *Pokémon* company to threaten to sue the researchers if they did not change the name. The gene is now more prosaically named as Zbtb7. However, some scientists have managed to name the genes for the arylsulfatase E as ARSE, the viral gene fuculokinase as fucK, and Poly (ADP-ribose) polymerase as PARP.

The important take-home message concerning our DNA, is that what defines us genetically is not how much DNA we have, or even how many genes; it is the complexity of how our genes are used and how these genes are controlled to interact with one another to carry out the various functions that give us our unique characteristics as humans.

# WHAT IS A MUTATION?

*We all carry genetic mutations that may place us at risk for future disease – therefore we are all at risk for discrimination.*

Bill Frist: A Senator Speaks Out on Ethics, Respect, And Compassion

There are no two genetically identical humans, aside from identical twins. On average, each of us is more than 99.9 per cent genetically identical to any other person. The less than 0.1 per cent of genetic variants distinguishing our genomes are present in different frequencies in different human populations.

DNA sequence variations are described either as mutations or polymorphisms. The difference between these two terms reflects how common they are; polymorphisms are more common and mutations rarer. A combination of the Greek words *poly* (multiple) and *morph* (form), a polymorphism describes multiple forms of a single gene (known as alleles) that exists in an individual or among a group of individuals. We have 2 copies of each gene, one from each parent, and so can have 2 different alleles. Polymorphisms differing by a single nucleotide, referred to as Single Nucleotide Polymorphisms (SNPs), occur about once every 1000 base pairs in the genome. Many SNPs occur in genes and in their surrounding regions important in controlling their expression. The effect of a single SNP on a gene may not be large - perhaps influencing the activity of the encoded protein in a subtle way - but even small effects can influence susceptibility to common diseases, such as heart disease or

Alzheimer's disease. Different SNPs vary in frequencies between different populations. As such, a very rare disease allele in one population can be classified as a mutation but as a polymorphism in another population if it is in a higher frequency. A good example is a SNP that causes the disease sickle-cell anaemia. In Caucasian populations, this is a rare sequence variant of the beta-globin gene that causes this blood disorder. In certain parts of Africa, however, the same allele can be described as a polymorphism as it is more common. The reason for this is that it confers some resistance to the blood-borne parasite causing malaria, that is more prevalent in parts of Africa. Another example is a polymorphism in the acetaldehyde dehydrogenase gene (ALDH) that produces an enzyme to convert acetaldehyde to acetic acid as part of our body's metabolism of alcohol. This polymorphism changes the structure of the enzyme making it less able to do this job, so rendering an individual more sensitive to alcohol; people with this DNA sequence develop red flushes, headaches and nausea when drinking alcohol due to the build-up of higher levels of toxic acetaldehyde that cannot be metabolised further. Around half of Asian ancestry have inherited this gene variant, while it is rarer in Caucasians.

Metabolism of alcohol (ethanol) to acetaldehyde and then acetic acid

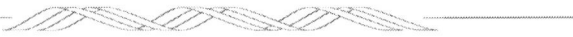

# WHAT IS A CHROMOSOME?

*For each chromosome contributed by the sperm, there is a corresponding chromosome contributed by the egg; there are two of each kind, which together constitutes a pair.*

Thomas Hunt Morgan

If all the 3 billion base pairs of DNA in a single cell of ours were laid out it would span 2 meters in length. If the entire DNA from the roughly 30 trillion cells that make up our body were joined together – about 60 billion kilometres – it would form a tiny stretch of nucleotides that would stretch to Pluto and back 5 times. This 2 meters of DNA needs to fit into a nucleus of around 6 micrometres (i.e. 6000th of a meter) diameter – a size

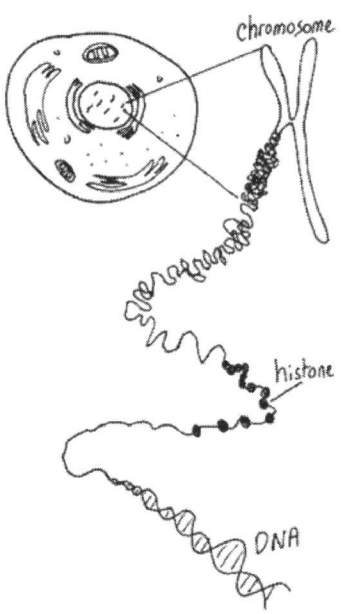

DNA wraps around histones to form chromosomes that are found in the cell

14

approximately a third of a million times smaller. To allow this huge mass of DNA to fit into a relatively small cell, it is packaged. It is twisted, folded and wrapped around proteins, called histones, into much more compact structures, known as chromosomes. At 5 micrometres long these chromosomes allow tens of thousands-folds reductions in length! A chromosome is, therefore, a strand of DNA wrapped around specific proteins that is found in the nucleus of eukaryotic cells.

Different species have characteristic numbers of chromosome pairs, known as a karyotype (Gr. *Karyon*; nut, referring to the nucleus). Mice have 20 pairs of chromosomes, dogs 39, fruit flies 8, some ant species only 2 and some crayfish species have 200 chromosomes! Needless to say, the number of chromosomes in an organism bears little relation to the complexity of the organism.

Humans have 23 pairs of chromosomes. It was a laboratory accident with a dilute salt solution that swelled cells causing the chromosomes to separate sufficiently to allow an accurate count in 1956 - over a century after chromosomes were first observed. These 23 pairs are found in each cell of our body, except red blood cells that do not contain a nucleus, and also some outer skin cells. Gametes, describing eggs and sperm, carry only one copy of each of the 23 chromosomes. These single copies then combine at fertilisation to give a total of 23 pairs again. In 1971, at a conference in Paris, our human chromosomes were numerically named from 1 to 22 according to their size, and referred to as autosomes. The 23rd pair of chromosomes were called 'X' and 'Y' and termed the sex chromosomes-males generally have an X and a Y chromosome, while genetic females usually have two X chromosomes. This scheme of coding chromosomes is still in use today, though in making the original assessments of size a mistake was made – chromosome 22 is actually longer than chromosome 21 and so the numbers should have been reversed.

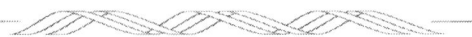

# WHAT IS A PROTEIN?

*The amino acid sequence of any protein is determined by the sequence of bases in some region of a particular nucleic acid molecule.*

Francis Crick

The word "protein" was introduced into science by the Swedish chemist Jons Jacob Berzelius (1779-1848) (Gr. *proto*; of primary importance). Proteins are made up of hundreds or thousands of smaller units called amino acids, which are attached to one another in long chains. There are 20 different types of amino acids, including Alanine, Aspartic acid, Leucine etc., that can be combined to make a protein. The sequence of amino acids determines each protein's unique 3-dimensional structure and its specific function. The order of amino acids in any protein is determined by the base sequence of nucleotides in the DNA coding for the protein, i.e. a gene. Three sequential nucleotides, called a codon, can encode one amino acid. As there are 4 bases, taken three at a time, this gives 64

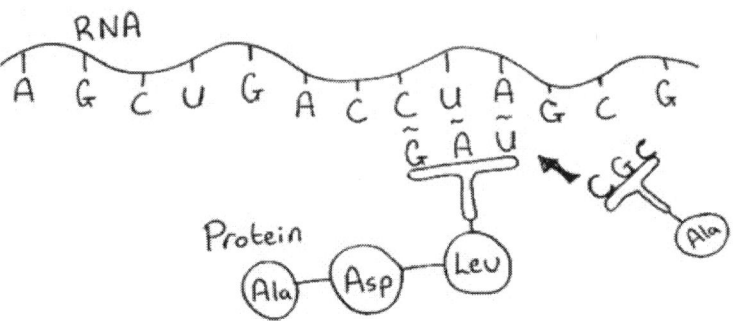

Translation of RNA to protein

combinations; since there are only 20 amino acids, there is more than one codon per amino acid, in most cases. There are also codons that signal the start and end of a protein. RNA is "read" to produce a sequence of amino acids making up a protein using adaptor molecules, called tRNAs, that have an amino acid at one end and at the other, an anticodon for matching a codon in the mRNA.

Proteins are required for the structure, function, and regulation of the body's cells, tissues, and organs. To do this, each protein has unique functions. Examples of proteins include whole classes of important molecules, among them enzymes, hormones, and antibodies. In 1955, the British double Nobel prize winner, Sir Frederick Sanger, was the first person to determine the complete amino acid sequence of a protein, insulin. His second Nobel prize was for developing a method to sequence DNA. The Sanger Institute in Cambridge, UK, bears his name and is one of the world's leading genetics research centres playing crucial roles in sequencing human genomes.

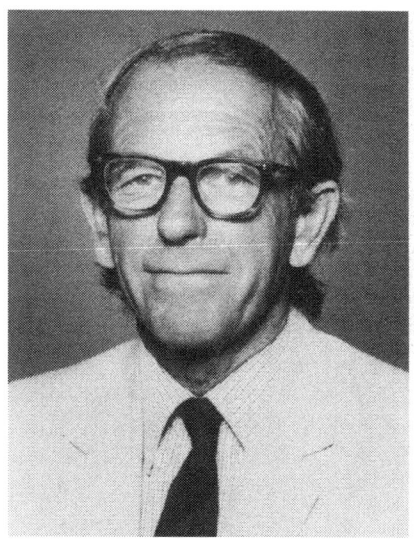

Frederich Sanger, 2006

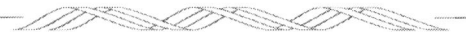

# GENETIC INHERITANCE

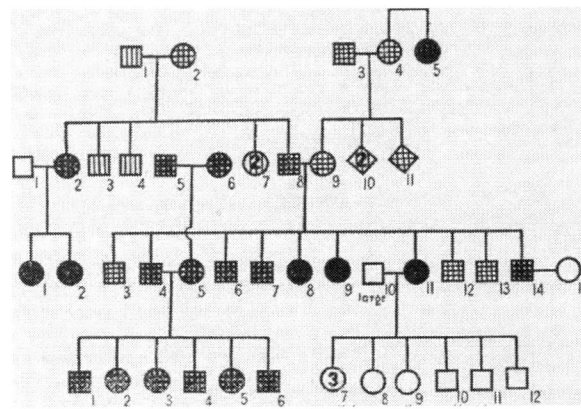

*We are machines for propagating DNA, and the propagation of DNA is a self-sustaining process. It is every living object's sole reason for living.*

Richard Dawkins

It was an Austrian Monk, called Gregor Mendel, in an Augustinian Abbey in Brno, the Czech Republic, who first laid down the laws of genetic inheritance. In the 1860s he noticed that if his pea plants producing purple flowers were pollinated by white-flowered

18

pea plants, the resulting seeds all produced plants with purple coloured flowers. If these purple-flowered offspring were then crossed together, a population (known as an F2 generation) of plants are produced in which three-quarters have purple flowers and one-quarter white flowers, i.e. a 3:1 ratio of purple to white.

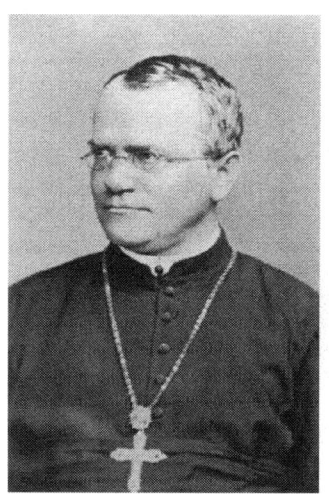

Gregor Mendel

From this data, Gregor Mendel developed the laws of genetic inheritance. When an organism has two different variants (we use the term alleles) for a trait, the allele that is expressed, overshadowing the expression of the other allele, is said to be dominant (i.e. the purple flower – denoted by allele P in the diagram). The gene whose expression is overshadowed is said to be recessive (i.e. the white flower – denoted by allele p).

Mendel published his findings in 1866 in the little-known journal *Proceedings of the Natural History Society of Brunn*. Arguably among the most exciting findings ever in the field of science, signalling the birth of genetics, his research initially had little impact being cited only three times over the next 35 years! His ideas and discoveries were simply too far ahead of their time and too contrary to popular beliefs about heredity. "*My time will come,*" he once said. It was not until 1900 that other scientists rediscovered his work; Hugo de Vries published similar results but neglected to mention Mendel. This prompted Carl Correns - a

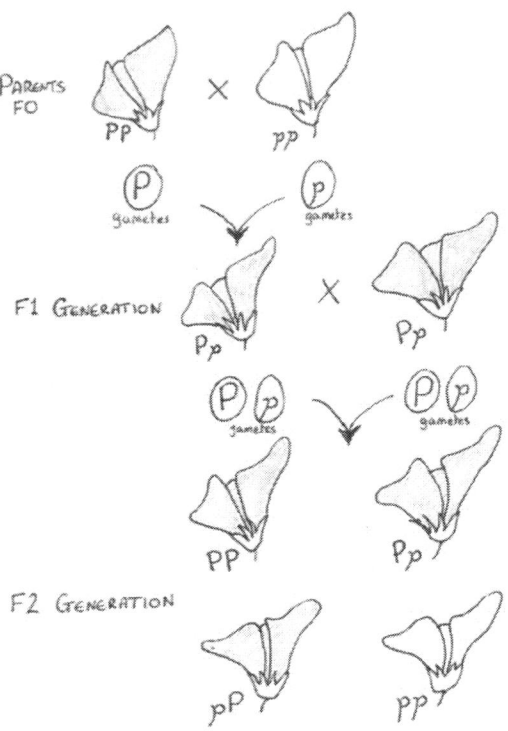

Inheritance of flower colour in pea plants

student of the renowned botanist Nägeli, with whom Mendel corresponded about his work with peas but who failed to understand its significance - to remind de Vries about Mendel. Coincidently, at the same time, Erich von Tschermak, the grandson of Mendel's old botany teacher, also produced supporting findings. However, Mendel had long since died in 1884 from kidney disease.

Why is this work so important and how does this inheritance of flower colour in pea plants relate to us? Sexual reproduction in humans, like plants, occurs with the fusing of two gametes. An oocyte and sperm, each with one-half of the pairs of 23 chromosomes, join together resulting in a cell and subsequent offspring inheriting one copy of a chromosome, with the respective genes, from each parent. When an identical mutated gene or allele is inherited from each of the two parents, the individual is referred to as homozygote for that allele as they have two copies of the same polymorphism or mutation. A heterozygote refers to the presence of only one copy of a particular allele.

A Mendelian trait or disease is, therefore, one that is controlled by a single allele (i.e. gene mutation or polymorphism) and shows a simple Mendelian inheritance pattern – either dominant or recessive, like the pea flowers. However, other patterns of inheritance occur if a gene is on the X chromosome (sex-linked) or mitochondrial DNA (mitochondrial inheritance). In addition, there are many disorders that involve several different genes, referred to as polygenic, or are influenced by other genes in combination with the environment, which are termed multifactorial and inherited in a non-Mendelian fashion.

# DOMINANT INHERITANCE

*I would rather make my name than inherit it.*

William Makepeace Thackeray

An example of a dominantly inherited trait can be seen in the presence of the Habsburg jaw in the family tree of the Habsburgs, one of the greatest royal houses of Europe. They passed on a gene for an inherited condition known as mandibular prognathism which, in mild forms, is relatively common and causes a jutting jaw or drooping lower lip: think of *Bubba Gump* or Jay Leno.

Parent 1: heterozygous (Habsburg jaw)

| Parent 2: Heterozygous (Habsburg jaw) | | H | h |
|---|---|---|---|
| | H | H/H (Habsburg jaw | H/h (Habsburg jaw |
| | h | H/h (Habsburg jaw | h/h (normal jaw) |

Parent 1: homozygous (Habsburg jaw)

| Parent 2: homozygous (normal jaw) | | H | H |
|---|---|---|---|
| | h | H/h (Habsburg jaw | H/h (Habsburg jaw |
| | h | H/h (Habsburg jaw | H/h (Habsburg jaw |

Parent 1: heterozygous (Habsburg jaw)

| Parent 2: homozygous (normal jaw) | | H | h |
|---|---|---|---|
| | h | H/H (Habsburg jaw | h/h (normal jaw) |
| | h | H/h (Habsburg jaw | h/h (normal jaw) |

Punnet squares showing inheritance of the Habsburg jaw

The presence of the protruding "Habsburg" jaw shows a pattern whereby the gene allele for the Habsburg jaw (H) is dominant over a normal shaped jaw (h). Therefore, individuals who are heterozygotes (H/h) inheriting both an allele for the Habsburg jaw and one for a normal jaw will nevertheless show the characteristic Habsburg jaw. If two heterozygous (H/h) parents produce children, there is a one in four chance of any of their offspring inheriting both attached alleles (h) and so having a normal jaw; the classic 3:1 ratio among offspring of heterozygous parents. This can be seen in the table above which is known as a Punnet square.

If one parent is homozygous for the Habsburg jaw allele (H/H), even if the other

22

parent has a normal jaw (h/h), then all children will have the Habsburg jaw, i.e. they will be heterozygotes (H/h). If both parents have normal jaws and are therefore homozygotes (h/h), then all offspring will have normal jaws also. However, if one parent is heterozygous (H/h) while the other has a normal jaw (h/h), then there is a 50% chance that any child will have a normal jaw or the Habsburg jaw, a 1:1 ratio.

The inherited characteristic of the Habsburg jaw or lip had been passed through generations of the family from as far back as 1421 when a jutting-jawed princess Zimburg

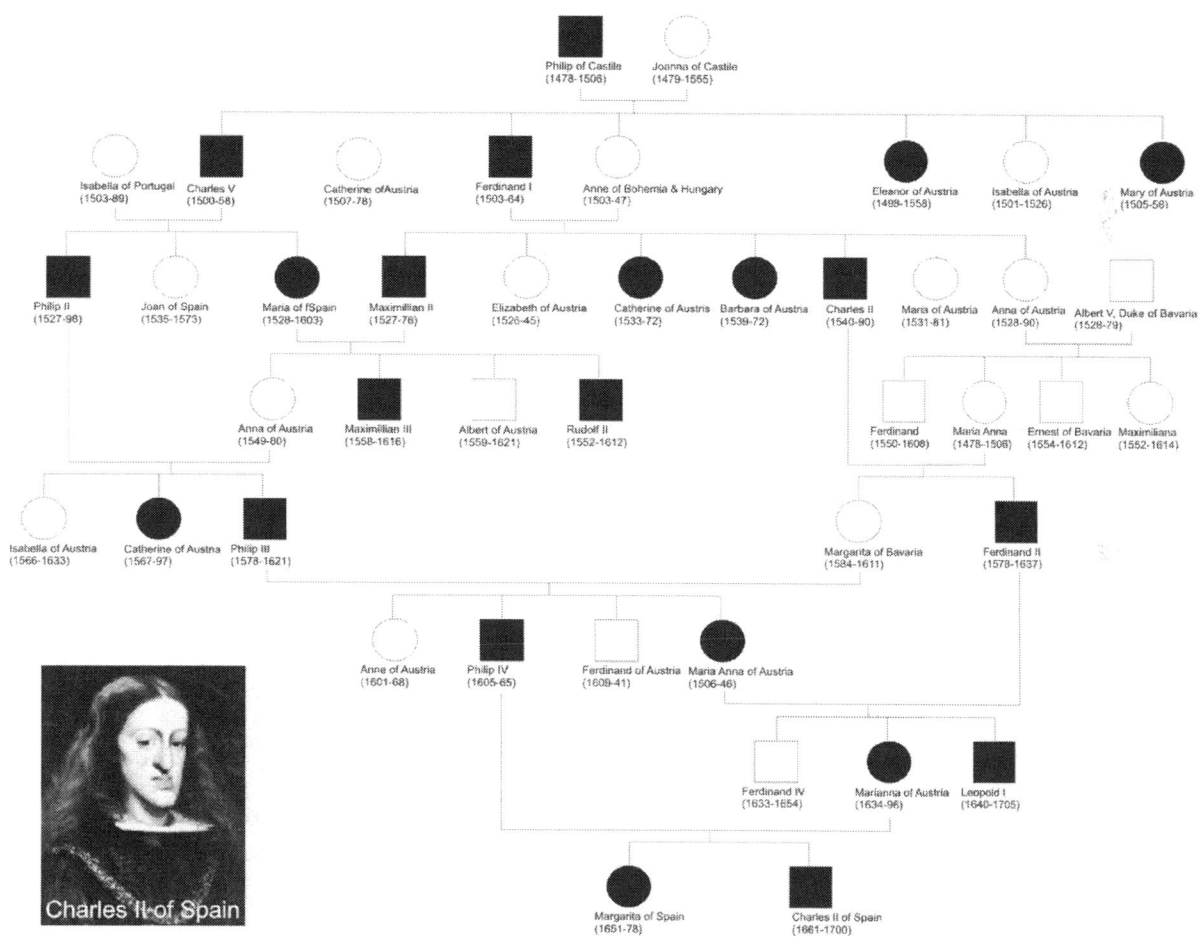

Inheritance of the Habsburg jaw, judging from portraits. Shaded boxes denote the presence of mandibular prothaganism in males (squares) and females (circles).

of Masovia married one of the Habsburg princes. For the next 300 years, the characteristic jaw would remain a defining feature of one of the greatest European dynasties. Indeed, it appears evident from portraits that members of the family were very keen to parade their under-bites as a mark of royalty. If we look at just the Spanish members of the Habsburgs, starting with the aptly named Philip 'the Handsome' and his wife Joanna 'the Mad' of Castile, it can be seen that both male and female members of the family at each generation were affected, ending with the unfortunate Charles II. Charles II's parents, who were uncle and niece, both appeared to have the Habsburg jaw and so possibly passed on a double dose of the gene to their son who was consequently born with a hugely misshapen jaw that prevented him from eating or speaking properly. Throughout his rule, he became increasingly mentally and physically decrepit and was unable to produce an heir to the Spanish throne. His eventual death led the War of the Spanish succession that would last for over a decade and involve much of Europe.

# RECESSIVE INHERITANCE

*Inbreeding is how we get championship horses.*

A Louisiana state representative, explaining why he was fighting a proposed anti-abortion bill that allowed abortion in cases of incest

Recessive inheritance can be thought of as the white flowers from Mendel's pea experiments. One example of recessive inheritance, sticking with royal families, can be seen in the appearance of earlobes. Some people have their earlobes hanging free, known as detached ear lobes, while others have the lobe attached to their head. This can be seen in the British Royal family, judging from photographs.

The inheritance of the ear lobe tends to show a pattern whereby the gene allele for detached earlobes (E) is dominant over attached (e). Therefore, heterozygotes containing both an allele for detached and one for attached earlobes have detached ears. And if two such heterozygous parents produce children, then there is one in four chance of any of their offspring inheriting both attached earlobe alleles and so showing attached earlobes; the

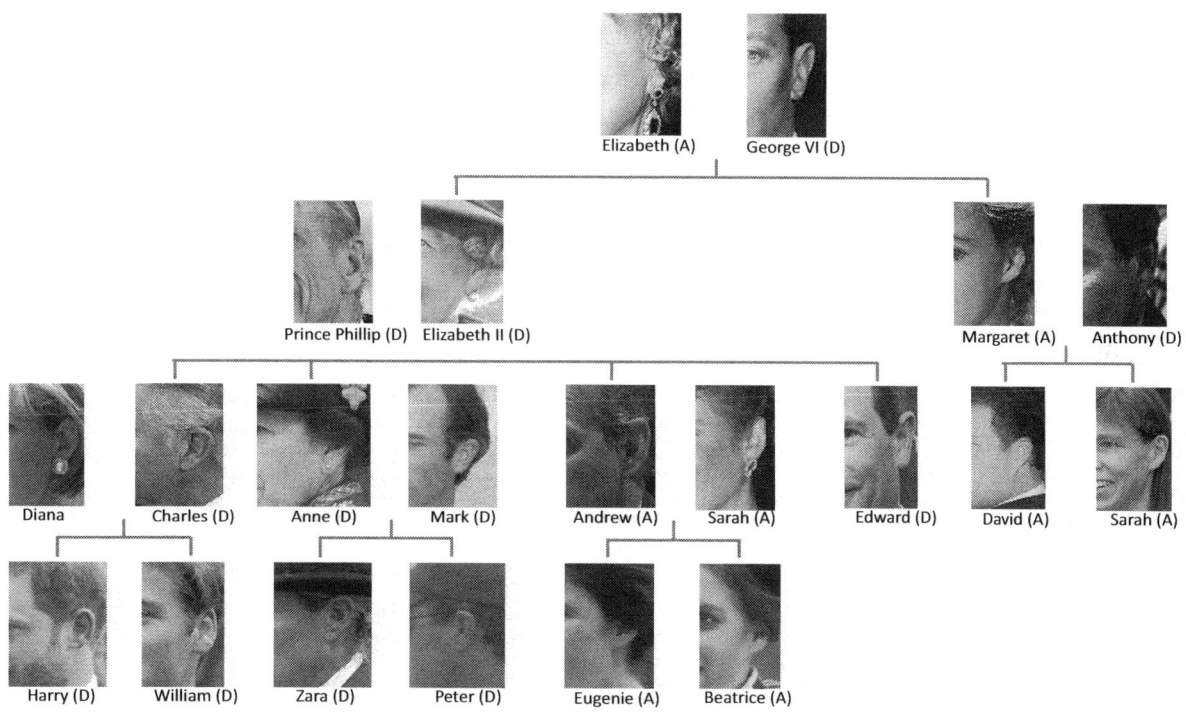

Inheritance of earlobe form in the British Royal family, judging from photographs. Names with boxed pictures denote the suspected presence of attached earlobes

classic 3:1 ratio.

Prince Andrew and Sarah Ferguson both seem to have attached ear lobes, suggesting that they are e/e, and as such their two daughters seem to have inherited the same trait. This would imply that both Queen Elizabeth (her sister Margaret had attached ear lobes) and the Duke of Edinburgh are heterozygotes (E/e), as one of their four children (Andrew) shows attached ear lobes. However, it should be stressed, like the Habsburg jaw, these are just examples of traits that seem to show a Mendelian inheritance pattern in these two families and is obviously not a means of testing paternity, and there is no identified gene for either.

Recessively inherited disorders occur in the same way, only resulting if two copies of the defective genes are inherited. Inheriting only one defective copy will not lead to any ill-effects as a second functional copy of the gene will compensate. So, while a dominant disease requires only one parent to carry the gene, a recessive disease can only result if both parents have at least one copy of the defective gene - 25% of the offspring of two such

Parent 1: heterozygous

| | | D | d |
|---|---|---|---|
| | D | D/D | D/d |
| Parent 2: Heterozygous | d | D/d | d/d (disease) |

Punnet square showing inheritance of a recessive disease-causing allele

heterozygous (i.e. they only carry one mutant copy of the gene) parents will show the disease. We can see this if we assume the dominant non-disease-causing gene as the 'D' and the recessive, disease-causing, gene as 'd'.

Therefore, in recessively inherited disorders the parents are often unwitting heterozygous carriers of a gene in which children inheriting two copies suffer from the disease. The family tree of a recessive gene is very different from a dominant one, as only one or two generations will suddenly show the disease when related individuals with the same disease-causing gene produce children.

The ancient taboo of incest in most cultures probably stems from the realisation that inbreeding, particularly within the first generation, leads to higher occurrences of children born with defects. The reason inbreeding is so detrimental to a population is that, while normally only a small minority of the general population will carry a copy of a particular gene causing a specific recessive disease, and hence the chance of meeting a carrier of the same recessive gene is low, this chance will increase if those individuals are related and hence share some genetic material. This explains why some recessively inherited conditions are found in higher frequencies in some close-knit communities such as Amish or various

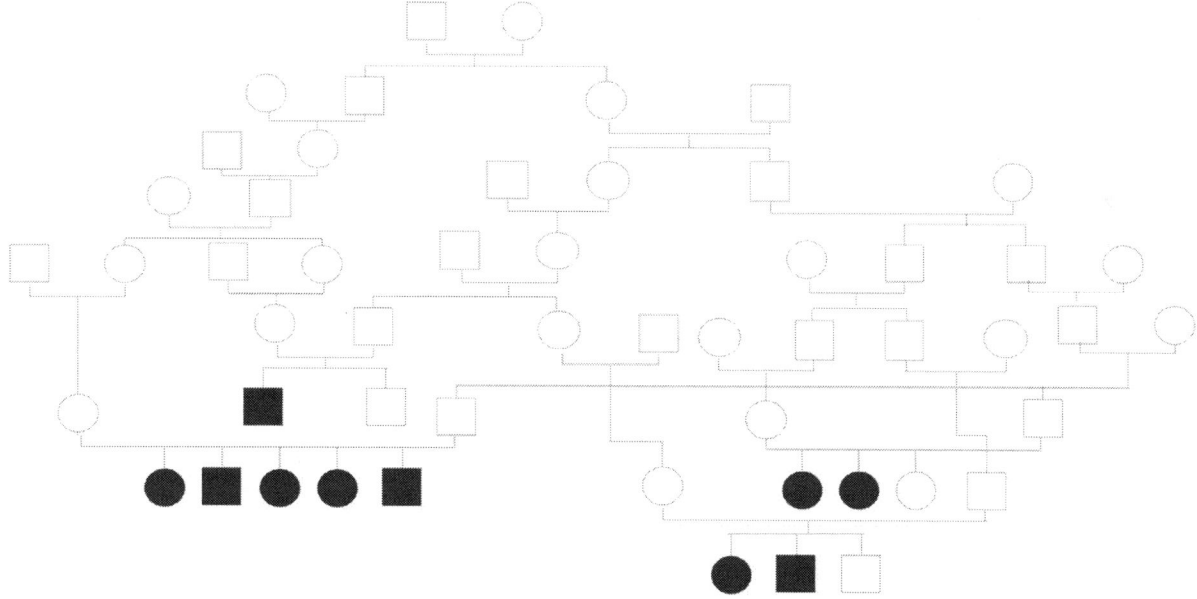

An example of inheritance of a recessive trait in males (square) and females (circle) in a family tree leading to a genetic disease (black). Notice how the affected individuals are all related.

Jewish communities. Another example of inbreeding leading to higher incidents of genetic diseases can be seen in the Negev Bedouin people, a population of 140,000 people who roam the Negev desert in Southern Israel. Their tradition is to marry within the family so as to strengthen bonds among extended families; over half marry their 1st or 2nd cousins. Though they may not carry any more mutations than the general population, as so many marry relatives, they have a higher chance of marrying someone carrying the same mutation. This increases the odds of producing a child with a recessive genetic disease. Consequently, many of the diseases commonly seen in the Bedouin are extremely rare in other populations around the world.

The French painter Henri de Toulouse-Lautrec was born from a first-cousin marriage with the recessively inherited bone disorder Pycnodysostosis. His parents must have both carried a copy of the mutated gene for the disease. At least three of his cousins, the offspring of his paternal uncle married to his maternal aunt, also suffered from the same disorder, supporting the mode of inheritance being autosomal recessive and highlighting again the risks of inbreeding.

Charles Darwin was among the first to realise the ill effects of inbreeding and the advantages of cross-breeding. In a letter to parliamentarian John Lubbock in 1870, he wrote "*consanguineous marriages lead to deafness and dumbness, blindness [etc.]*," and asked if the government could gather data about the frequency of cousins marrying and the health of their offspring. He nevertheless, himself married a cousin, Emma Wedgwood.

Consanguinity (Lat. *con*, together; *sanguis*, blood), in clinical genetics, is generally defined as a union between two individuals who are related as second cousins or closer. When it comes to consanguinity, it is difficult to beat the Ptolemies, the last dynasty of

Greek Egypt, who traditionally married brother and sister. The most famous, Cleopatra VII, was at different times married with two of her brothers (Ptolemy XIII and Ptolemy XIV) as well as having relationships and children with Julius Caesar and his most trusted general, Mark Anthony.

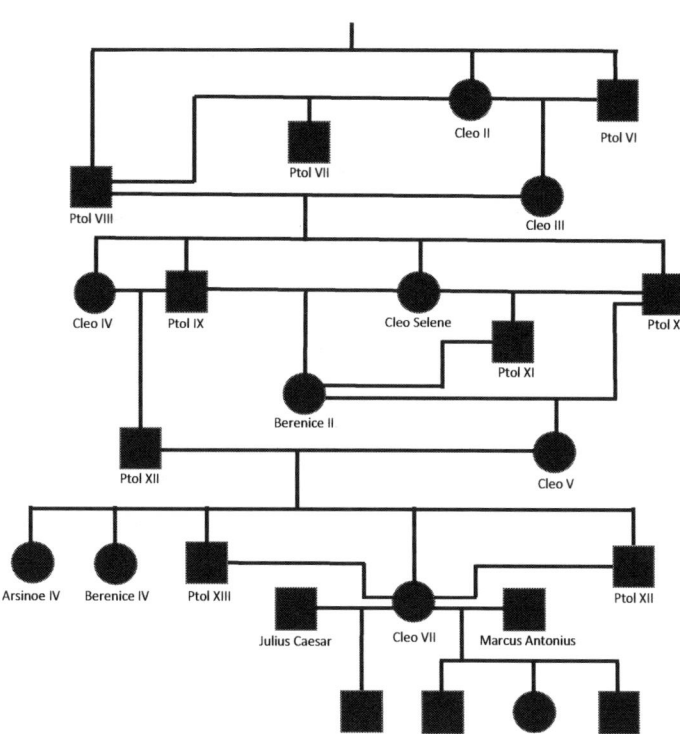

Part of the possible Ptolemaic genealogy. Cleo; Cleopatra, Ptol; Ptolemy.

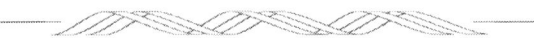

# SEX-LINKED INHERITANCE

*If no fresh blood is infused occasionally the races would degenerate physically and morally.*

Queen Victoria in 1885 writing concerning the proposed marriage of a granddaughter

When a gene for a genetic disease occurs on the X chromosome as opposed to one of the autosomes, X-linked recessive inheritance is seen (X-linked dominant inheritance is rarer). This inheritance is characterised by a high preponderance of male sufferers – in contrast to the inheritance of traits on autosomal chromosomes, where both sexes have the same probability of expressing the trait. The reason females are less affected by X-linked recessive diseases is due to the presence of two X chromosomes. They can carry the affected gene on one X chromosome without developing the disease but can pass it on to their sons and can hence act as unaffected heterozygous carriers. This can be seen in the inheritance of the X-linked recessive disease haemophilia, in the British royal family. Queen Victoria was almost certainly a heterozygous carrier of the haemophilia gene, which she passed on to one of her sons, Leopold, who subsequently suffered and died from the disease. Interestingly, Queen Victoria had no ancestors with the condition and so serves as an example of how a disease can arise due to a spontaneous mutation; however, there are suggestions that she may have been illegitimate. Prince Leopold then passed on his mother's gene to his daughter, Alice, who subsequently gave birth to a haemophilic son. Two more of Queen Victoria's children, her daughters Alice and Beatrice, also inherited

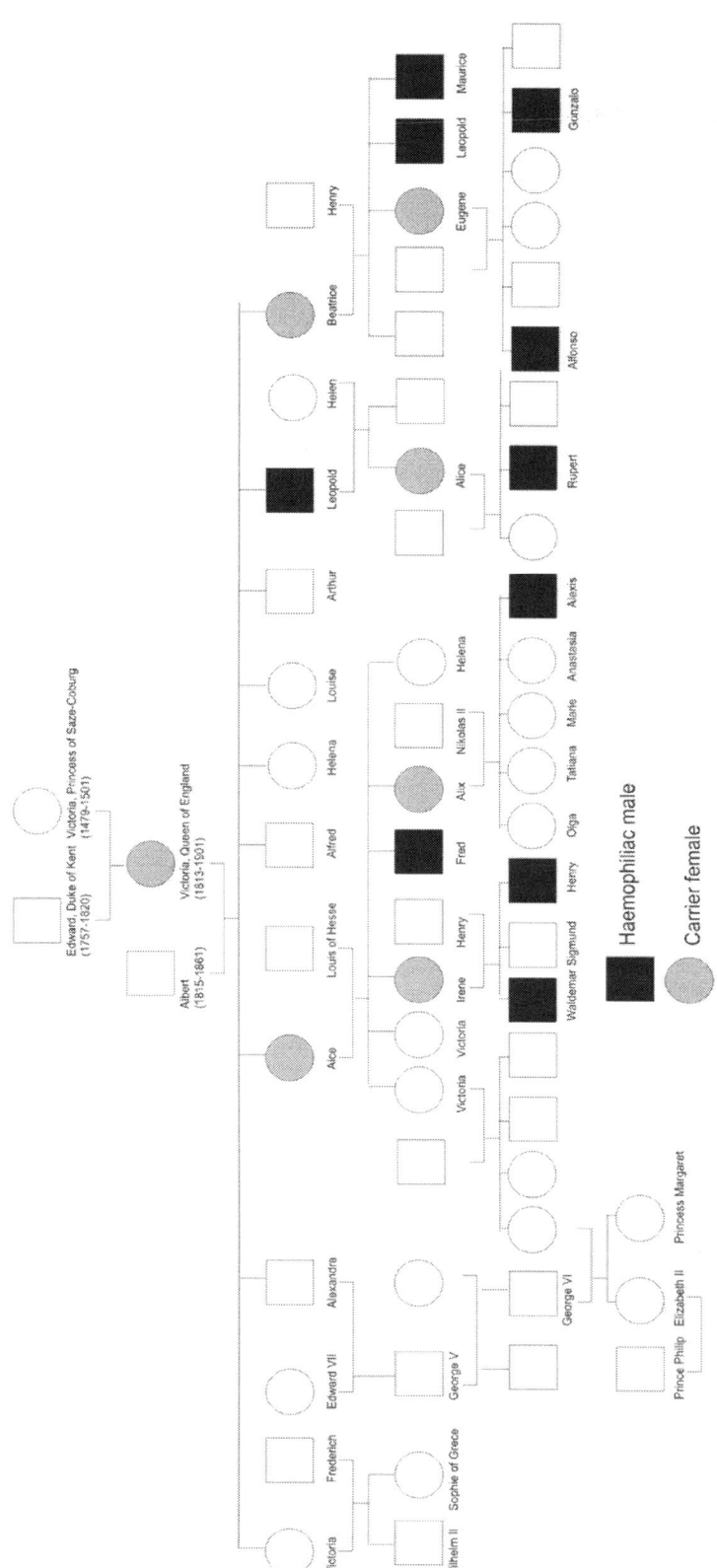

Family tree of the British and European Royal families showing the inheritance of haemophilia (black) in males (boxes) and females (circles).

The haemophilia gene acting as unaffected carriers. They, in turn, transmitted the genetic disease to several royal families in Europe, including Spain and, more famously, Russia with the birth of Alexis, the son of Tsar Nicholas II of Russia.

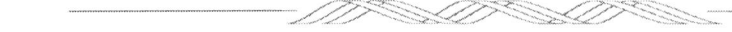

# MITOCHONDRIAL INHERITANCE

*All modern humans are related to what scientists call "Mitochondrial Eve." This refers to our common matrilineal ancestor. She lived approximately 200,000 years ago and depending on how you estimate the length of a generation, we are only 5,000 to 10,000 generations from one another. To put it another way, each of us is a cousin of one another at most 10,000 times removed. And yes, Mitochondrial Eve lived in Africa, so, in a very real way, we are all Africans.*

Desmond Tutu

Mitochondria are organelles, found in our cells, that produce energy. They contain their own DNA and divide independently of the cell. During sexual reproduction mitochondria are passed on to offspring only through the egg and not the sperm as it is only the nucleus of the sperm, which contains no mitochondria, that enters the egg during fertilisation. Thus, only females can pass on mitochondria. Consequently, only females can pass on mitochondrial diseases such as mitochondrial myopathies and Leber's congenital optic neuropathy, discussed later. That the mitochondrial DNA we carry in our cells has been carried through a direct line from our very distant maternal ancestors has formed the basis of the 'Eve Theory' in which all mitochondria present in the whole human population originate from a single, or a small handful of, women who lived around 100,000 years ago in Africa.

As polymorphisms or mutations within mitochondrial DNA are passed on only through females it is possible to determine to what extent individuals share the same maternal ancestor. This was used to test the late Russian imperial family and the fate of one of the Tsar Nicholas II's daughters, Anastasia. She was presumed executed along with the rest of her family on July 17, 1918. However, rumours spread that Anastasia might have survived, especially later when remains of two of the children were found to be missing from the rest of the Romanov's grave. In 1922 a woman, later called Anna Anderson, claimed to be Anastasia, and although she could not speak a word of Russian, many people

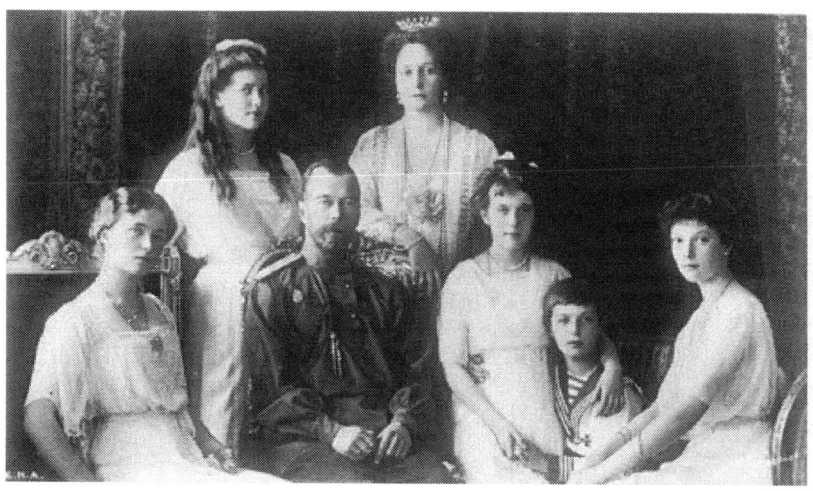

The family of tsar Nicholas II of Russia. Left to right: Grand Duchess Olga, Grand Duchess Maria, Nicholas II, Alexandra, Grand Duchess Anastasia, Tsarevich Alexei, Grand Duchess Tatiana. 1914

were convinced. To determine if her claims were true her mitochondrial DNA was taken from locks of her hair, found after Anna's death, and compared to mitochondrial DNA extracted from the bones of Anastasia's mother, the Czarina. As a control, mitochondrial DNA from England's Prince Philip, who is related on the maternal side to the Czarina, was compared to the Czarina and indeed showed significant relatedness. But Anna Anderson's mitochondrial DNA showed very little similarities to the Czarina's mitochondrial DNA, leading one to conclude that she was not Anastasia. However, further analysis of mitochondrial DNA from a grandnephew of a Polish factory worker, Franziska Schanzkowska, who disappeared at about the same time that Anna Anderson appeared in Germany claiming to be Anastasia, revealed strong similarities, suggesting this as her real identity. In the summer of 2007, a second grave was discovered with the remains of two children that further mitochondrial DNA testing revealed to be Alexei and one of his sisters, presumably Anastasia.

# MULTIFACTORIAL INHERITANCE

*I got a hundred bucks says my baby beats Pete's baby. I just think genetics are in my favour.*

Andre Agassi, married to Steffi Graff, referring to Pete Sampras who is married to a non-grand slam winning-tennis player, actress Bridgette Wilson.

Some disorders, such as haemophilia, cystic fibrosis and sickle cell anaemia (all described later), are caused by mutations in a single gene, known as monogenic (Gr. *mono*, one). These show clear Mendelian inheritance patterns such as autosomal dominant or autosomal recessive, or X-linked. Other disorders, can either be caused by one gene or multiple genes (polygenic) or exhibit a complex inheritance. Common medical problems such as heart disease, type 2 diabetes, and obesity generally do not have a single genetic cause but result from multiple genes together with lifestyle and environmental factors such as diet and lack of exercise. Known as complex or multifactorial disorders, these conditions may tend to "run in families" but do not show dominant, recessive, sex-lined or mitochondrial inheritance patterns. Many other traits such as height, skin colour, intelligence and personality also result from a complex constellation of genes. For example, a recent study comparing DNA differences from over 240,000 people in the UK found 538 gene variations linked to intellectual ability. But, even with all these genes, it was still only possible to predict 7 per cent of a person's intelligence. As it is thought that over half of our variation in general intelligence is due to genes, there must be many more to be discovered, perhaps in specific combinations. Environment plays an important role too. For example, well-nourished children brought up in safe, unpolluted and stimulating environments score better in IQ tests than deprived children. It is being able to control for these environmental differences that make finding genes for complex disorders, complicated.

Epilepsy is an example of a group of common neurological disorders characterised by great variation in severity and inheritance, being multifactorial and involving the influence of multiple gene variants. Within the Roman Julio-Claudian dynasty, there are descriptions of epilepsy, amongst other neurological conditions, in a number of the emperors and family members that are not clearly Mendelianly inherited through each generation.

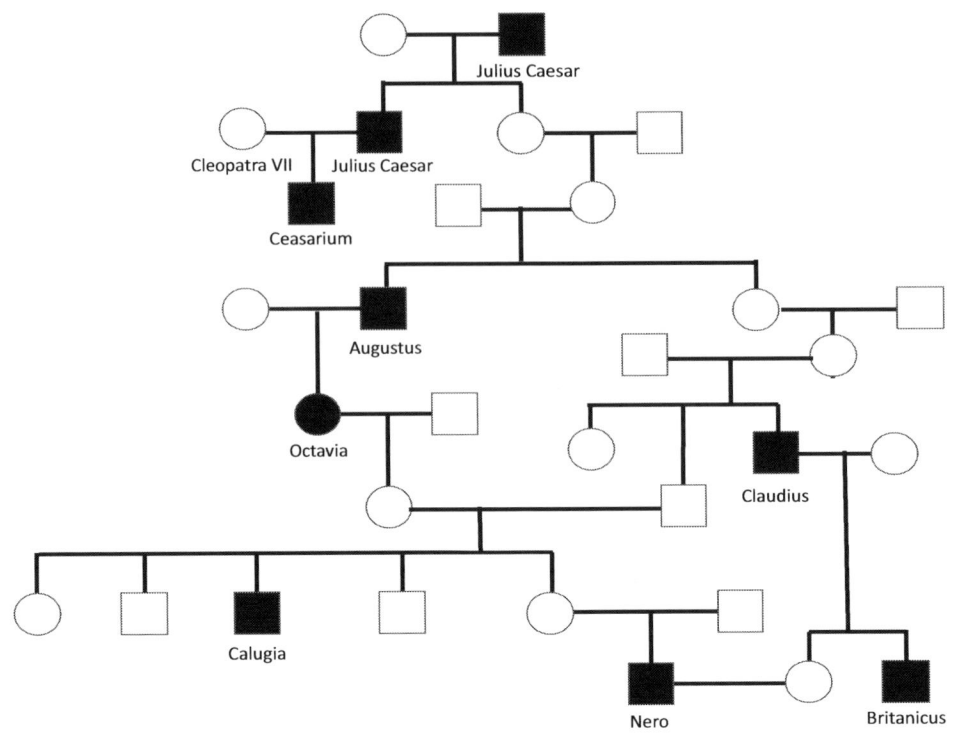

A highly simplistic version of part of the Julio-Claudian family tree focusing on only those members suggested to have suffered epilepsy (shaded shapes).

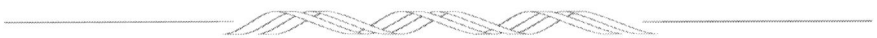

# EPIGENETICS

*Epigenetics has always been all the weird and wonderful things that cannot be explained by genetics.*

Denise Barlow

Epigenetics (Gr. epi, above) is the study of changes in gene regulation independent of DNA sequence. The term was coined by C. H. Waddington in 1942 to describe the differentiation of cells during development. For example, it explains how a skin cell and a neuron have the same DNA sequence but obviously perform very different jobs.

One function of epigenetics is to imprint some genes dependent from which parent they derive. This phenomenon of epigenetic imprinting, that a set of chromosomes would behave differently if coming from either the mother or the father, though only relatively recently understood at the molecular level, has been known since ancient times. For instance, this can be seen in the old practice of producing mules. A female horse needs to be mated with a male donkey to produce a mule; an animal prized for its very hardy temperament. In contrast, mating a male horse with a female donkey produces an animal known as a hinny. Smaller than a mule with a head more similar to a horse, a hinny has less strength, stamina and hardiness than a mule - definitively not the animal you want for carrying heavy loads around. Mules have been described in Egypt since before 3000 BC. George Washington, was a keen mule breeder and, after begging the King of Spain, was

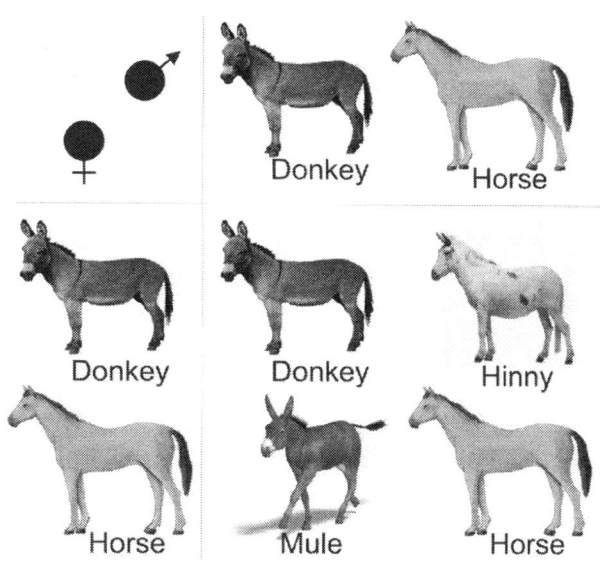

A male donkey crossed with a female horse gives a mule while a
female donkey crossed with a male horse gives a hinny

37

eventually rewarded with a huge male Catalonian donkey, called the *Royal Gift*. This amazing animal was used to sire many mules and generally considered as the father of the mule industry in the United States, upon which much of America was shaped and built.

Epigenetic imprinting is, therefore, able to explain how a foetus of any mammal cannot develop when both sets of chromosomes come from the same parent. This is because a small number of particular genes are epigenetically modified and expressed according to their parent of origin, either on the maternal or the paternally inherited chromosome. This means that a foetus inheriting two maternal sets of chromosomes will have twice the normal expression of some imprinted genes that are only expressed on the maternal chromosomes and a complete lack of proteins that would normally be expressed from the paternal chromosome – such a scenario is not compatible with life.

While only a small percentage of our genes are imprinted, mutations affecting one of these will lead to disorders which differ depending on whether the gene defect was inherited from the mother or father. For example, an individual missing a small piece of chromosome 15 from the mother has a disorder known as Angelman syndrome. In contrast, if the abnormal chromosome 15 is inherited from the father the offspring will present with Prader-Willi syndrome characterised by lower IQ, small stature and a tendency for overeating that can lead to obesity later in life. Such individuals might steal and hide food, like the fictional *Billy Bunter*. Katie Price's eldest son, Harvey, suffers from this disorder, in addition to the blindness disorder septo-optic dysplasia, which she has commented causes him to want to continuously eat and even steal food if nobody is looking.

The physician Harry Angelman, first described Angelman syndrome in 1965. It was while he was on holiday in Verona that he happened to see Giovanni Francesco Caroto's painting, *Boy with a Puppet*. The boy's happy expression and the jerky movement of the puppet of which he holds a picture, reminded Angelman of some of the behaviours of three young patients back in his paediatric ward in Warrington, UK. This included other characteristics of the disorder with frequent laughter and smiling, often with little stimulus and being easily excitable, often accompanied by flapping of hands. He originally used the now-defunct name of *"Happy Puppet Syndrome"*. Colin Farrell has spoken of this disorder that affects his eldest son, James adding *"Be careful of judging what your child is capable of. You have to watch your child and give him every opportunity to see how they respond. Let your child decide what his limitations are."*

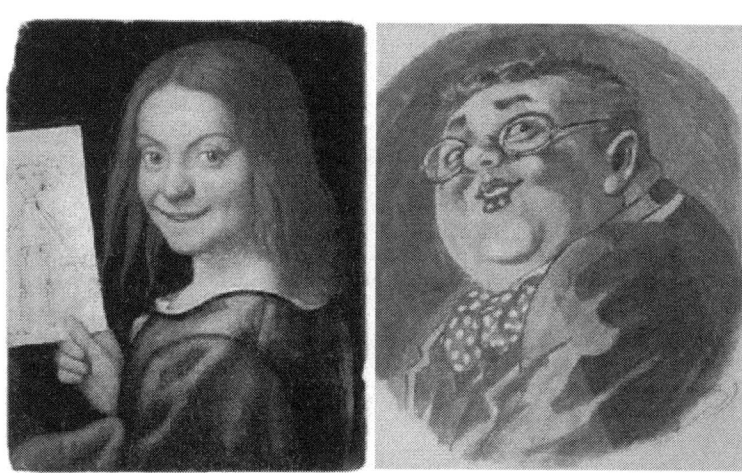

*Boy with a puppet*, Giovanni Francesco Caroto (1480–1555). Billy bunter by C. H. Chapman

The molecular mechanisms for how epigenetics works is complex and involves modifications of the DNA and chromatin but not the basic sequence of DNA. This can play a role in what has come to be known as cell memory as a genome can add and remove epigenetic marks, controlling specific genes, in response to various stimuli. In this way an organism can regulate its genes long after the stimulus has passed allowing it to quickly adapt to an environment. There is the hypothesis of Developmental Origins of Disease in which early exposure to an environment can program later risk for disease. An example is seen in the Dutch Hunger Winter famine during November 1944 as a Nazi barricade during World War II, resulted in a severe famine and starvation that lasted until spring of 1945. Individuals who were in utero during this time were subject to different outcomes depending on the period of time in which they were conceived: those who were in the 1st trimester during the famine were likely to be born normal size, but with higher risks for developing high blood pressure, diabetes, and obesity. Those who were in the 3rd trimester during the famine, were born small and remained smaller in adulthood without any higher risk for obesity or diabetes.

The actress, Audrey Hepburn, was a teenager during the famine and was extremely malnourished. Surviving on a diet of dug-up tulip bulbs and salad leaves, she weighed 40kg by the time the war ended, aged 16. She often commented how she believed this permanently affected the rest of her physical and mental health, suffering from edema, jaundice, anaemia, respiratory illnesses, and unable to put on much weight.

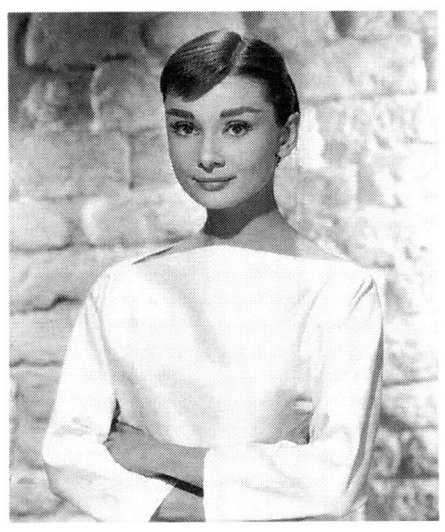

Audrey Hepburn, 1956

# POPULATION GENETICS

*I have called this principle, by which each slight variation, if useful, is preserved, by the term of Natural Selection.*

Charles Darwin

A number of genetic disorders occur more frequently in certain ethnic populations. For example, one in 27 individuals within the Ashkenazi Jewish population carry the recessive allele for the severe genetic disorder Tay-Sachs Disease, a disorder that is very rare in the general population. Likewise, within Amish communities, there are an unusually high proportion of people with certain specific genetic conditions such as Ellis-van Creveld syndrome. Although again extremely rare globally, affecting around 1 in 150,000 people worldwide, Ellis-van Creveld occurs in 1 in 5,000 individuals within Pennsylvanian Amish populations. Both these are described later.

Mutations or polymorphisms lead to variant forms of a gene. These different gene forms are known as alleles and they may lead to an individual being born with a genetic disease. If the allele behaves dominantly or recessively will determine if an individual will need to inherit, respectively, only one copy of the defective allele from one of the parents, or two copies - one form each parent - to develop a disease. All recessively inherited disorders occur when affected individuals inherit a defective allele from each parent. Those with only one copy of the abnormal allele experience no symptoms of the disorder. In seeming contradiction, some disease-causing alleles can actually confer a benefit to an individual. One of the most well-known examples is the gene polymorphism for sickle cell anaemia; this results in a devastating disease in individuals with two copies of the allele, but shows some protection against malaria in individuals who only inherit one copy. In human populations plagued with a high presence of malaria, such as in Africa, the sickle cell allele has therefore remained in the gene pool, by being selected for through resistance to malaria.

Population genetics is the study of such genetic variation within populations to try to understand mechanisms behind the changes in frequencies of genes and alleles in populations over space and time.

Reginald Punnett was a research fellow at Cambridge in 1900 when Mendel's work was rediscovered. He had the original article translated into English and set about repeating and building on these experiments working on chickens and peas. In order to predict the probability of possible genotypes in offspring, he created the Punnet square. This was used to schematically explain the ear lobes of the royal family in the previous chapter. For example, in the punnet square shown, two heterozygous (E/e) parents with detached earlobes have a 3 in 4 chance of producing children with detached earlobes, the dominant trait (E/E, E/e, e/E), and 1 in 4 children with attached, the recessive trait (e/e). In 1908, following an astute question from a student during a lecture, he further wondered how a dominant gene allele would not become fixed and pervasive in a population and a harmful recessive version would not simply disappear over time. In other words, if a healthy gene were dominant over the other allele that caused a genetic disease, why would those diseases still be present in the population? He explained this problem to his cricketing partner and mathematician, Godfrey Hardy, who a few months later published what came to be called Hardy's Law, and then Hardy-Weinberg equation when it was realised that German physician Wilhelm Weinberg had figured out and published the same rule a few months earlier.

The equation states that the amount of genetic variation in a population will remain constant from one generation to the next (in the absence of disturbing factors, that we will discuss shortly). We can use two hypothetical gene alleles, "A" and "a", to explain the Hardy-Weinberg equation: $p^2 + 2pq + q^2 = 1$. In a population, p is the frequency of "A" and q is the frequency of "a". Therefore, $p^2$ represents the frequency of the homozygous genotype "AA", $q^2$ represents the frequency of the homozygous genotype "aa", and 2pq represents the frequency of the heterozygous genotype "Aa". The sum of the allele frequencies for all the alleles must be 1, so $p + q = 1$. If the p and q allele frequencies are known, then this equation can be used to calculate the frequencies of the three genotypes.

Why is this important? For example, the latest figures in the UK show 1 in every 2,500 babies is born with the recessive condition cystic fibrosis and so this is the number of homozygous cystic fibrosis allele carriers. Therefore, $q^2$ is 1/2500 and q is 1/50. For the

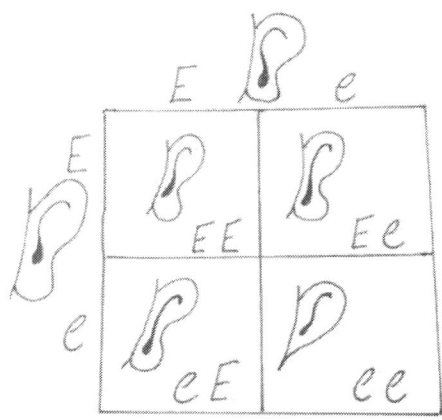

A Punnet square showing the inheritance of earlobe form

43

non-disease-causing allele p is 49/50. You can then calculate the proportion of heterozygous carriers of the disease allele 2pq is 2x (1/50 x 49/50) = 0.0392. This means that, out of every 100 people, 3.9 of these on average are heterozygous carriers of the cystic fibrosis allele. This is crucial information when advising couples in family planning. The UK government also use this information to legislate routine testing of all infants for this disease, as part of the heel-prick blood test in new-borns.

The Hardy-Weinberg equation can be also used to measure whether the observed genotype frequencies in a population differ from the frequencies predicted by the equation. Because populations are always evolving, frequencies of alleles do not stay the same for long as there are always forces acting upon them. For example, there are new mutations and natural selection, and also the phenomena of gene flow and genetic drift.

Natural Selection occurs when one allele confers some benefit to the individuals that bear it and is thus favoured by natural selection over time. Remember the advantage conferred to an individual having one copy of the sickle-cell anaemia allele, concerning malaria. This violates Hardy-Weinberg Equilibrium because the frequency of the beneficial allele will increase over time. The opposite will be true for an allele that harms the individuals who inherit it, the frequency of which will decline over time until it is eliminated.

Gene Flow refers to the movement of genes or alleles into or out of a gene pool. This can happen when members of a population migrate out, or members of another population migrate in and interbreed. For example, sickle cell anaemia is the fastest-growing genetic disease in the UK. Most cases worldwide are in sub-Saharan Africa but migration of people to the UK has led to an increase of this disease, so much so that all new-borns in the UK are tested for this disorder as part of the hell-prick test. A recent study showed that the mutation for this disease first occurred 7,300 years ago in one child born within the Bantu population of West Africa.

Genetic Drift refers to changes in gene frequencies due to random events, which can happen very quickly, producing dramatic and sudden effects. Drift can occur when a small group becomes isolated from the larger population. This is often called the Founder Effect. Drift can also occur when a catastrophic event reduces a large population to a very small size, known as a bottleneck. Genetic drift means that the gene pool shrinks and becomes less diverse, which is often the opposite of what happens during gene flow when interbreeding expands the gene pool and increases genetic diversity.

A Founder effect describes the loss of genetic variation that occurs when a new

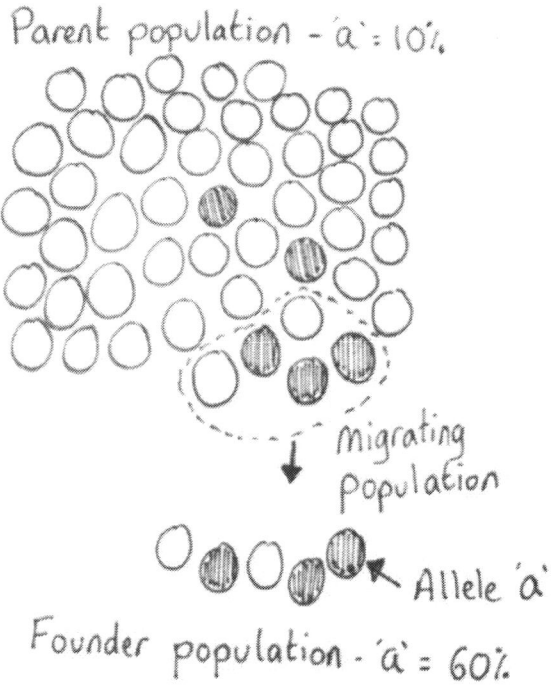

A founder effect is where a small number of a population carrying a disproportionate frequency of alleles forms a new population

population is established by a very small number of individuals from a larger population. This type of genetic drift is experienced by some Amish communities descended from a small group of around 200 people who left their roots in Germany to travel to Pennsylvania. By chance, one or two of the individuals, carried the Ellis-van Creveld gene allele leading to a higher frequency of this than the larger population from which they came. When they became the founders of the new population of Amish in America, their descendants also exhibited this higher frequency.

If you imagine a bottle containing a gene pool, then the neck of a bottle allows just a small fraction of the gene pool out. When a population suffers a sudden catastrophic decline and is then repopulated by a small group of survivors, a bottleneck event occurs.

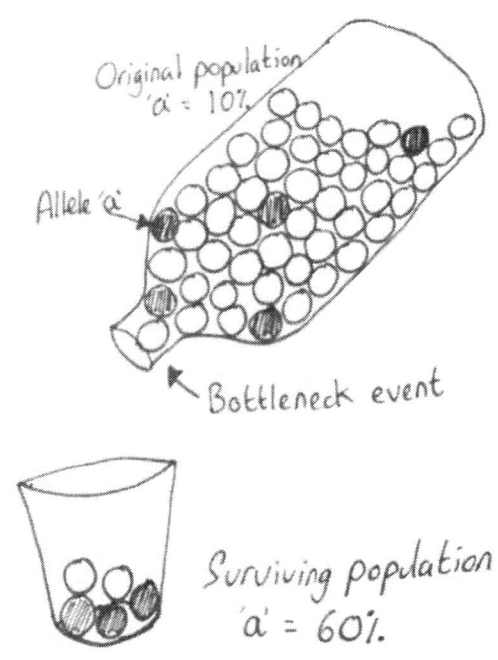

A diagram to show how a bottleneck can quickly change frequencies of genes within a population

The gene pool shrinks and the new frequency of alleles for each gene are different from what it was in the larger population prior to the event. In this way, previously rare alleles

46

can suddenly become common, purely by chance. This happens in nature all the time. On the island of Pingelap, in the Pacific Ocean, up to 1 in 10 of the population are born totally colour-blind due to inheriting the autosomal recessive disorder achromatopsia (Gr. *a*, without; *chroma*, colour; *opsia*, optic/sight). A further 30 per cent are unaffected carriers. In the global population and the UK, only around 1 in 30,000 individuals are affected. This high prevalence on the island has been traced back to a population bottleneck in 1775 following a tsunami that swept through the island killing all but 20 inhabitants. One of survivors included the ruler, Doahkaesa Mwanenihsed, who is believed to have been a carrier for this genetic condition. Inter-breeding between the descendants of his have since resulted in the higher frequency of the recessive allele and presence of this disorder. But why have the affected individuals not been selected against leading to a reduction in this high frequency? There is some suggestion that Pingelapese sea-fisherman with this condition, though having difficulty seeing in bright sunlight, have better vision at night, seeing in much fainter light than people with normal vision can; a trait that could be useful for night fishing.

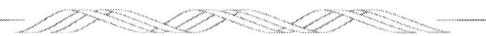

# CHROMOSOMAL DISORDERS

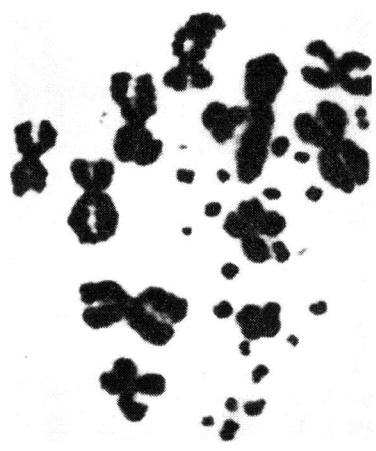

*One chromosome too many to be declared a woman for the purposes of athletic competition*

International Association of Athletics Federations disqualifying Ewa Klobukowska from competition in 1967.

Chromosomal disorders can result from changes in either the number or structure of chromosomes. Changes in the number of chromosomes happen when there are more or fewer copies of a particular chromosome than usual. Changes in chromosome structure

48

happen when the material in an individual chromosome is missing, disrupted or rearranged in some way.

We usually have 23 pairs of chromosomes giving a total of 46. Some people though are born with either too many or too few chromosomes. As a cell gets ready to divide, chromosomes are separated into each of the dividing cells by proteins that bind and physically separate them. A failure of this during the production of sperm or oocytes can result in these cells lacking or gaining a chromosome. Following fertilisation this can produce an offspring, containing only a single chromosome or three chromosomes instead of the usual pair.

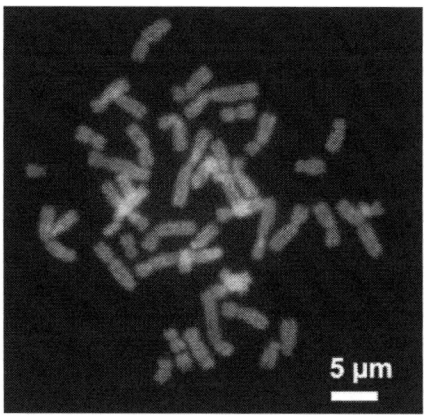

Human chromosomes

These numerical chromosomal abnormalities tend to occur more in females during the production of oocytes with increasing age. It is thought that as the molecular apparatus involved in separating chromosomes in older oocytes cells ages so mistakes in chromosome separation occur. Men on the other hand constantly produce new sperm throughout their lives. This explains why the risk of producing children with numerical chromosome disorders, such as Down's syndrome, is higher in older women.

Chromosomal abnormalities occur in around 1 in 200 births and account for around half of all miscarriages. Although extra numbers of any chromosome can occur, only extra copies of the X and Y chromosomes (Klinefelter's, Triple X and XYY syndromes), and chromosome 21 (Down's syndrome) are able to survive past infanthood. Children born with three of chromosome 18 (Edwards Syndrome or 13 (Patau Syndrome) are born with severe developmental defects and often do not survive for more than a year. A foetus lacking any chromosome of a pair, apart from the X chromosome, known as Turner's syndrome, is unable to survive to survive to birth.

One of the most common examples of a disorder caused by an extra chromosome is Down syndrome. People with this condition have 47 chromosomes in their cells instead of 46, due to three copies of chromosome number 21 instead of the usual pair. The extra set of genes on chromosome 21 lead to increased levels of certain proteins that can result in risks of hearing and vision defects, heart abnormalities and a range of developmental difficulties involving delayed coordination skills and mental abilities such as speech and short-term memory. Though people with Down's syndrome share some common physical and mental characteristics, this will be different for each person and they will have different personalities and abilities. With good support and healthcare, many people with Down's syndrome can leave home, have relationships, work, and lead largely independent lives.

Born in 1996, the Australian model Madelaine Stuart has been described as the world's first professional model with Down syndrome. Heart defects are very common in people with Down's syndrome and Madelaine, at only a few weeks old had major heart surgery, and again aged 21. People with Down syndrome also tend to have a lower metabolism that can increase risk for weight gain. Though Madeline struggled with her weight for a long time, it was following a change in diet and fitness that her photo shoots started to go viral and is she is changing society's perception of people with disabilities, one photo at a time. She has appeared on the New York Fashion Week catwalk, Paris fashion week, London fashion week, and numerous more and named Model of the year for 2016 by World Fashion Media. With calls for more diversity Madelaine has developed a marketing campaign endorsing numerous products and has established her own Fashion Label: *21 Reasons Why by Madeline Stuart.*

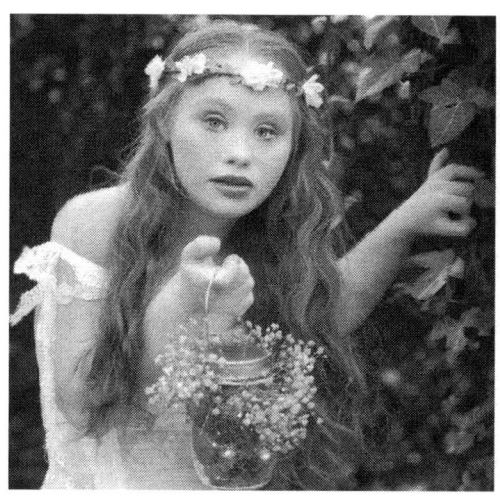

Madelaine Stuart

Chris Burke, best known for his role as Corky Thatcher in the *TV series Life Goes On,* became the first person with Down syndrome to star in a weekly television series. The British actor, Tommy Jessop, is the first actor with Down syndrome to star in a prime-time BBC drama, *Coming Down the Mountain*; a performance that was widely praised and helped earn a BAFTA nomination. Jessop made his television debut in *Holby City,* and has also appeared in *Casualty, Monroe* and *Doctors,* and played *Terry Boyle* in series 5 of *Line of Duty.* In March 2011 William Loughnane, 26, from County Clare, become the first person with Down's Syndrome to pass a driving test in Ireland, needing just five lessons and passing the first time.

Males normally inherit an X and a Y chromosome while females normally have two X chromosomes. As females possess two X chromosomes, they have two copies of every gene on the X chromosome while males only have one. This might mean that females could produce twice the amount of protein from these genes, on the X chromosome, then males. To balance this, females maintain only a single active X chromosome in each cell, while the second X chromosome becomes inactivated. This inactivated X chromosome is referred to as a Barr body and different cells randomly inactivate either of the two X chromosomes, so it is not the same X chromosome activated in every cell. However, not all genes on the second X-chromosome are inactivated; a few genes that are also found on the, very gene-sparse, Y chromosome escape inactivation.

In 2009, *The Daily Mail* reported a male Calico cat that its owners had named *Eddie*. These rare male Calico cats highlight both the importance of a Y chromosome for male sex determination and the process of X-inactivation. These black, ginger and white Calico cats are normally females because the gene for fur colour, containing a black and a ginger allele, is on the X chromosome. Therefore, only a female with two X chromosomes and the two

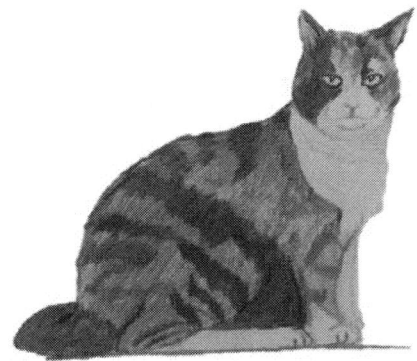

A calico cat

different alleles for the colours can produce the calico colour patterning; the patches of ginger and black depending on which X chromosome is active in those cells. For example, if the X chromosome carrying the black colour gene is inactivated, then the skin there will produce the ginger colour from the active X chromosome. The rare male calico cats highlight that the presence of two X chromosomes does not lead to femaleness; they have an XXY sex chromosome karyotype (Karyotype is a term to describe the numbers of chromosomes) and demonstrate that it is a copy of a Y chromosome that is needed to determine maleness. The name *Eddie* was therefore in homage to Eddie Izzard, essentially a male with a female coat.

Individuals inheriting only a single copy of a sex chromosome of a pair, i.e. the X chromosome, have Turner syndrome, a condition affecting about 1 in every 2,000 individuals. Having fewer copies of those few genes on the missing X chromosome, some of which drive bone growth, these women are usually shorter in stature, though growth hormone treatment is generally given to correct this, and may have a webbed neck that can be corrected with surgery. These individuals also tend to fail to develop secondary sex characteristics during puberty, which is again generally treated with oestrogen hormone therapy. Women with Turner's syndrome generally have underdeveloped ovaries and so tend to be infertile, though there is a wide range of symptoms and characteristics that can vary between individuals. Missy Marlowe, who is 155 cm tall, is a 1988 Olympic gymnast and 1987 Pan-American Games gold medallist, and spokesperson for the Turner Syndrome Society.

The inheritance of multiple X chromosomes can result in a female with a disorder known as triple-X. Having more X chromosome gene copies, especially those coding for bone growth, leads to taller than average height with unusually long legs and slender torsos. Found in around 1 in 1000 females it is relatively common. Many cases go undiagnosed as some women with the condition do not experience any or only mild symptoms. However, others may show developmental delays and learning disabilities.

The inheritance of an extra Y chromosome is known as XYY syndrome. These males generally have higher levels of testosterone owing to the extra Y that can sometimes result in severe facial acne during adolescence and increased height. However, most people appear physically and mentally normal and are often completely unaware of their condition. Occurring in around 1 in 1,000 males, a small percentage of these men are infertile, as the increased testosterone and other hormones can inhibit sperm production. Stefan Kiszko, who was jailed for the murder of 11-year-old Lesley Molseed in Manchester in 1975, had XYY syndrome. In an appalling miscarriage of justice, he spent 16 years in prison before he was released, after evidence showed that his semen samples contained no sperm, in contrast to the sperm found on Lesley Molseed's clothes. This sperm from the crime scene then provided DNA that was subsequently used to provide the evidence that finally helped to identify and convict the real murderer who is currently serving a life sentence for the crime. Stefan Kiszko, however, sadly died within a year of his release from a heart attack.

It is still often suggested that the high testosterone levels in XYY men can make them more prone to violence and criminal activity. Much of this stems from some completely discredited studies between 1965 and 1968. Around this time was the murder trial for Richard Speck who raped and brutally murdered 8 nurses in a Chicago dormitory. His lawyer argued that his acne and aggressive behaviour was proof of XYY and therefore he could not be considered legally responsible for his uncontrollable urges. Nevertheless, he was sentenced to life in prison where he eventually died. Amazingly, a chromosome test conducted during the trial that showed him to be normal XY was completely overlooked in the confusion of the courtroom drama. This idea of a link between XYY and criminality was used as the basis of the television fiction series *The XYY Man* about an individual with XYY, and thereby a natural criminal. The *Alien 3* movie also used this theme, being set in an off-world penal colony for prisoners with XYY. Needless to say, again, scientific evidence shows that a person with XYY syndrome is no more likely to commit a crime.

Individuals who inherit more than one X chromosome but still possess a Y chromosome are males who have what is known as Klinefelter syndrome (XXY). This is the same genotype as those rare male Calico cats. Affecting around 1 in 660 males in the UK, this leads to increased height from the extra chromosome and some feminine body contours, reduced facial and body hair, and lower testosterone levels. Generally, most appear normal physically and mentally with many again being unaware they have this extra chromosome. Some, however, may have problems with fertility. It should also be noted that people with Klinefelter syndrome are not more inclined to be homosexual, although a small number may be transgendered. The artist Lili Elbe was thought to have had this disorder. He married Gerda Gottlieb, one of the most influential Art Deco artists of the early twentieth century, and cross-dressed for her when she needed a female model.

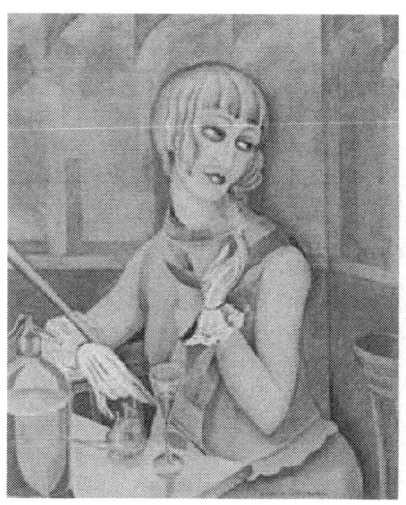

Lili Elbe by Gerda Gottlieb

He soon became Gerda's favourite model. It is interesting to consider to what extent the 1920's small-breasted feminine ideal may have been influenced by Lili's figure. Whilst undergoing a series of sex reassignment surgeries she died in 1931. Her story is now a major movie, *The Danish Girl*, starring Eddie Redmayne as Lili.

Inheriting more than two X chromosomes along with a Y chromosome results in karyotypes such as XXXY, which are still considered forms of Klinefelter syndrome. This is the chromosomal arrangement of Caroline Cossey, also known as Tula, who appeared in *the James Bond* movie *The Spy Who Loved Me*. Raised as a boy, she opted to live as a girl at a young age, undergoing sex-assignment surgery and subsequently becoming a well-known model and actress.

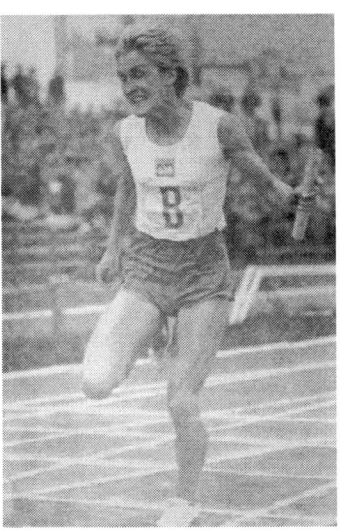

Ewa Klobukowska, 1964

Some people contain multiple different genotypes within their bodies, a phenomenon known as mosaicism. Though we develop from a single fertilised egg, defects can occur in early cell divisions with a result that two or more genetically different cell lines develop within a body. One lady with this anomaly was Ewa Klobukowska, a 1964

Olympic sprint bronze medallist who was the first woman to fail the sex chromosome test. It was during the 1967 European Cup, that the Athletics governing body told her and the world that she had failed the test, "*One chromosome too many to be declared a woman for the purposes of athletic competition*", and to return all her medals. She gave birth to a baby boy the following year. Later genetic testing revealed that she was a genetic mosaic of XX/XXY. Her humiliation led to massive changes in gender verification policies.

Changes in chromosome structure happen when the material in an individual chromosome is disrupted or rearranged in some way. A part of a chromosome can also become lost or deleted. This can happen with any chromosome, and if the missing region contains important genes, the individual may show impairments, a learning disability or other health problems depending on how much of the chromosome has been deleted, and where the deletion is. A chromosome may duplicate part of itself so that an individual contains too much of a particular chromosome region and the genes found within. Again, developmental problems may occur depending on which genes are impacted by this duplication and produce too much of those specific proteins.

One example of a loss of a part of a chromosome is Williams syndrome. Occurring in around 1 in 20,000 people, individuals inherit a chromosome 7 missing a region containing several genes which, when lost, lead to cardiovascular problems and a generally lower IQ. However, people with this disorder often show a great aptitude in language and music; many have near-perfect music pitch and a great sense of rhythm. Another characteristic of William's syndrome are 'elfin-like' facial features with a small upturned nose, depressed nasal bridge and a broad mouth with full lips. This, together with their often remarkable musical and verbal abilities, and highly sociable depositions, has led to the suggestion that affected children may have been the inspiration for folktales and legends such as pixies, elves and fairies, who were often musicians and storytellers.

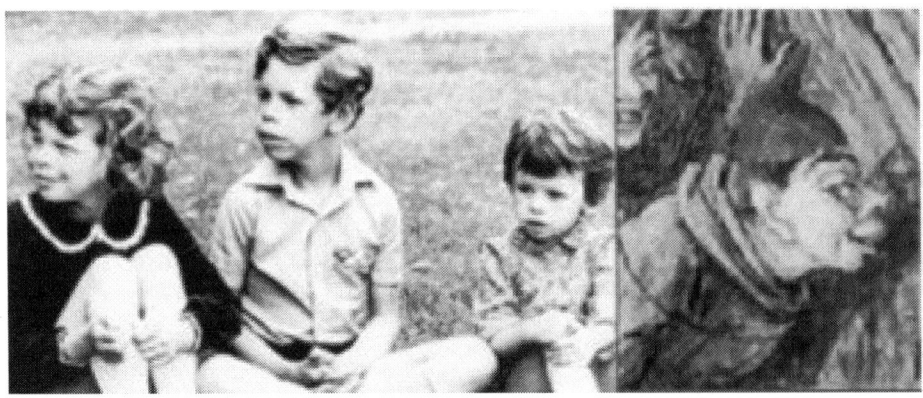

Unrelated children with Williams syndrome. An illustration of an elf by Richard Doyle

In some cases, one part of a chromosome can move and attach to a different part of the same chromosome or another chromosome or two pieces from two different chromosomes may swap. Known as translocations, the effect these have on the individual depends on whether any DNA has been lost or gained or if the DNA is differently active in another chromosome. This piece of a chromosome might disrupt a gene or may contain genes which, when moved to another chromosome, become more or less active leading to different amounts of protein. This occurs, for example, when a specific part of chromosome 8 containing the c-Myc gene is transferred (i.e. translocated) to chromosome 14 resulting in a change in the amount of a protein important in controlling cell growth and proliferation and so leading to Burkitt's lymphoma. This is a B-cell lymphoma, first described in 1956 by the British surgeon Dennis Burkitt whilst in equatorial Africa.

Interestingly, many of us carry "balanced" translocations with no obvious effect. There are theories that these balanced translocations may be important steps in speciation where genomes diverge to an extent that fertile offspring may no longer develop from a mating between two groups.

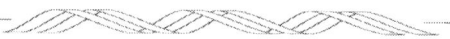

# SKELETAL DISORDERS

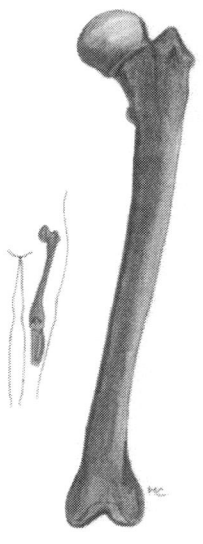

*My parents armed me with an amazing sense of humour, and it's what you need when, well, it's what anyone needs in this world*

Warwick Davis

Bone is living tissue performing many functions as well as providing mechanical support for the body. It is composed of a hard matrix of elements including calcium and potassium deposited around protein fibres such as collagen. In the developing foetus, the skeleton is first laid down as cartilage that is then replaced by bone. X-rays, especially in young children, will still show areas of cartilage present at the ends of growing bones; this can be used to estimate a child's age. However, even in adulthood, the size and shape of bones change and are continuously being remodelled in response to everyday stresses. In fact, the entire human skeleton is replaced every 10 years, through the activities of bone-dissolving and bone-rebuilding cells.

Skeletal defects are common birth abnormalities and can be caused by a variety of different genes leading to more than 200 distinct diseases. Genetic diseases can lead to reduced bone growth, increased bone growth or uncontrolled bone growth.

Diseases leading to reduced bone growth can lead to disproportionate short-stature: this differs from proportionate short stature such as seen in growth hormone deficiency. Depending upon which bones are primarily affected, such as in the limbs, trunk, or ribs, it is possible to differentiate by sight some of the various types of disproportionate short-stature, and in some cases which gene might be involved. One example is achondroplasia (Gr. *a*, lack of; *chondro*, cartilage; *plasia*, growth). This results from mutations in a gene that codes for a factor important in allowing cartilage cells to respond to growth signals during development. Cartilage makes up much of the skeleton during early development and is later converted to bone, except for the cartilage covering and protecting the ends of our bones and in the nose and ears. In achondroplasia, these cartilage cells develop into bone more slowly and this particularly impacts those quicker growing long bones of the arms and legs, leading to these becoming shorter. Slower growing bones within the body trunk, hands and skull tend to be of normal size. Interestingly, though this disorder is an autosomal dominantly inherited disorder, affecting around 1 in 25,000, many affected individuals are born to parents of average height. These cases represent new, sporadic, mutations that may be transmitted through the parent's germ cells, particularly the father's sperm. As men age their sperm accumulate more mutations resulting in a slight increase in the risk of fathering children with any kind of genetic disorder related to mutations.

Born to average-sized parents, and with an average-sized brother, *Game of Thrones* star Peter Dinklage, has this condition, as has Jason '*Wee Man*' Acuña the star of *Jackass* and a professional skateboarder. From the discovery of numerous mummified bodies and skeletons and statues, it appears that achondroplasia was unusually common in

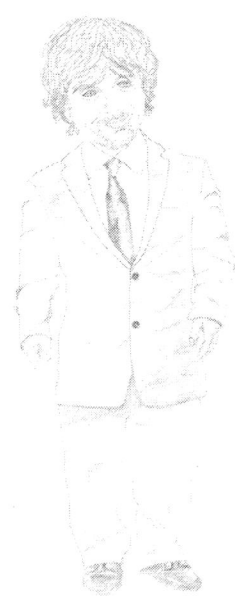

Peter Dinklage

ancient Egypt suggesting a total acceptance of this disorder in society, allowing individuals with the condition to marry without prejudice. There are two Egyptian gods, *Bes* and *Ptah*, that are often depicted as having a stature characteristic of this disorder.

Shimshon Ovitz was born in Romania in 1868 with a condition of short stature that he passed on to seven of his ten children, who were subsequently born with the disorder, all standing less than 3 feet tall. These individuals had disorder related to achondroplasia, called pseudoachondroplasia (Gr. *pseudo*, false). Though, somewhat similar in appearance this is an entirely separate disorder resulting from a mutation in a different gene coding a protein essential for the normal development of cartilage and its conversion to bone. Disruption of this protein means it is unable to do its proper job and instead levels of it build up inside the cartilage-forming cells leading to the cell's death. This, therefore, prevents normal bone growth, again particularly in the faster-growing long bones. The Ovitz family toured central Europe with this condition as entertainers known as *The Lilliput Troupe*. However, in May 1944 they were all sent to Auschwitz but were saved from the gas chambers by Josef Mengele for the purpose of experimenting on them. Working for his

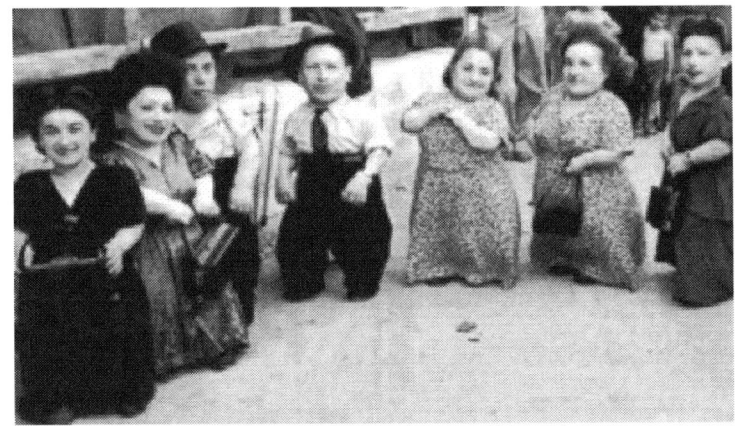

The Ovitz family arriving in Israel, 1949

mentor, Professor Otmar von Verschuer, he was interested in twins, and also dwarfism. They were subjected to various cruel and bizarre experiments until liberated by Russian troops. Amazingly, nearly all of them survived and the family made a new home in Israel where they once again became successful performers. Meanwhile, Mengle had escaped to Brazil, while Professor von Verschuer received the prestigious honour of the chair of human genetics at the University of Münster; a position he held until his death in a car accident in 1965.

Cartilage-hair hypoplasia (Gr. *hypo*, reduced; *plasia*, growth) is characterised by shortened arms and legs, small hands and a bell-shaped chest. Head size is usually normal with very fine sparse hair and individuals generally have immune defects that can lead to recurrent infections. This autosomal recessively inherited disease results from mutations in a gene important in regulating mitochondria in producing energy for cells and for processes involved in cell division and growth. Though generally rare, it is most common among the genetically isolated Amish population with around 1 or 2 in every 1000 born with the disorder. The late actor and star of the *Austin Powers* films Verne Troyer had this disorder, born to average-sized parents who were Amish. At 2ft 8in (81 cm) tall, actor Verne Troyer was one of the smallest actors in the movies. Sadly, suffering from depression and

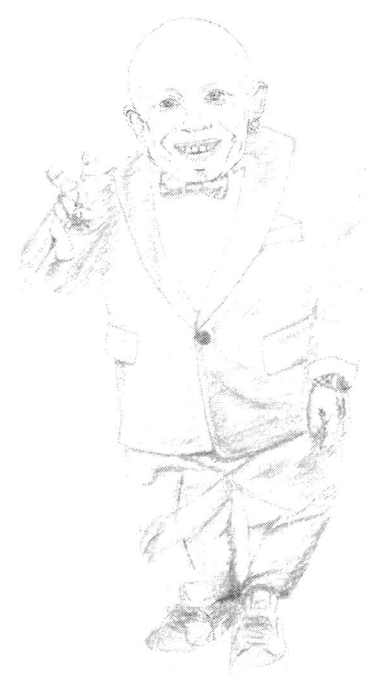

Verne Troyer

alcoholism he died in 2018 aged 49. The well-known American actor Billy Barty, who founded the organisation and charity *Little People of America,* was also born with this condition. His wife Shirly had a different short stature, Multiple Epiphyseal Dysplasia. Neither of their children had their short stature supporting the autosomal recessive inheritance pattern.

Warwick Davis, best known as *Professor Flitwick* in the *Harry Potter* movies and as *Wicket* in *Star Wars,* was born with a type of short stature disorder known as spondyloepiphyseal dysplasia congenita (*spondylo,* spine; *epiphyseal,* growing bones; *dysplasia,* abnormal growth; *congenita,* present at birth). This is characterised by a shortened body trunk, in addition to shortened arms and legs while the head, hands and feet are normal sized. This rare autosomal dominantly inherited disorder is caused by defects in a gene coding for a type of collagen protein, the main component of bone and cartilage, leading to reduced growth in the long bones and spine. Born to average-sized parents it would seem

Warwick Davis

he inherited a sporadic mutation in the gene that his two children also have. In 2012 he co-founded the charity *Little People UK* with a number of people including his wife Samantha who has achondroplasia.

In the late 1930s, two doctors, Richard Ellis and Simon van Creveld happened to share the same train compartment on the way to a paediatrics conference in England. After talking, they realised they each had a patient with similar characteristics including short stature with shortened arms and legs and ribs with a small chest together with the presence of more than the normal number of fingers or toes, known as polydactyly. Subsequently known as Ellis-van-Creveld syndrome, this disease results from mutations in either of two genes that have important roles in cell signalling. Cell-to-cell signalling allows cells to coordinate their activities, ensuring that tissues, organs, and systems function correctly and that also during development cells grow and form specific cell types important during development. Though relatively rare, this recessive disorder again has a very high incidence in the Amish, particularly those of Lancaster County, Pennsylvania where around 1 in every 200 are born with this. As described, this is an example of a founder effect as this

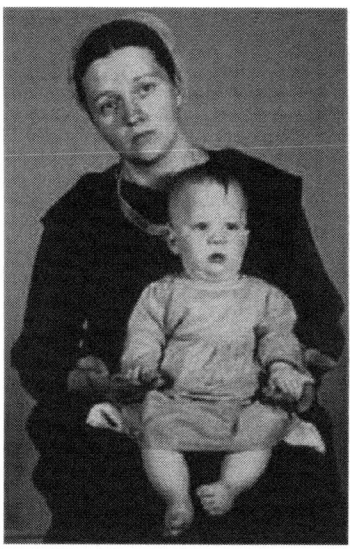

Ellis-van-Crevald syndrome in an Amish child

rather closed population stems from a small number of around 200 immigrants, including Samuel King and his wife who came to the area in 1744; one of these two must have carried a gene defect for the disorder. The well-known picture shown is of one of the descendants of this couple with her affected child.

Born in 1864 in San Carlos, Mexico, Lucia Zárate, has the Guinness World Record of being the lightest woman ever lived, at just 4.7lb, and one of the shortest at 21.5 inches tall. The calf of her leg was not much thicker as an adult thumb. She was the first person described with a type of primodial dwarfism; a term used to define someone with a smaller body size in all stages of life beginning from before birth. There are five different types that all show very short stature with a body that is proportionately formed, but very small. Most cases involve a disruption in skeletal growth or hormones but are not due to a deficiency of growth hormone, as in pituitary dwarfism. A number of different mutant genes have been found for the different types, many impairing cell division leading to reduced cell production and growth. Lucía Zárate made her debut at the Philadelphia Centennial Exhibition of 1876 and performed in various side shows, singing and dancing. It was whilst

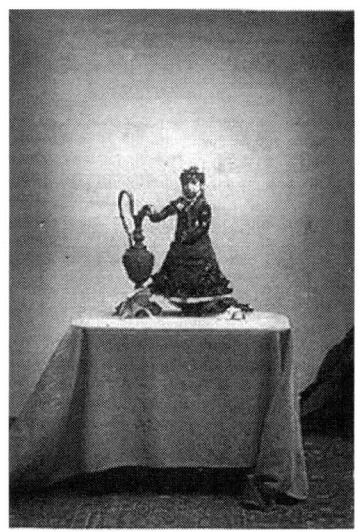

Lucia Zarate, 1890

exhibiting herself around the U.S. she died of hypothermia, aged 26, when the circus train she was travelling in became stranded in snow in the Sierra Nevada Mountains.

Some diseases result from gene defects leading to increased production of bone or cartilage. This can cause bones to become very brittle hence the name osteopetrosis (Gr. *osteo*; bone, *petros*; stone) given to these types of disorders. A mild type of this disorder is Albers-Schönberg disease characterised by weakened bones and deafness from mild bone overgrowth in the skull compressing nerves important for hearing. The American artist Laurel Burch had this disorder, suffering more than 100 bone fractures in her life before her death in 2007, aged 61.

Another disorder resulting in dense bones is pycnodysostosis (Gr. *pyknos*; dense, *dysostosis*; abnormal bone formation) resulting in disproportionate short stature. In this autosomal recessive disease, a mutation leads to a deficiency of an important enzyme found in cells called osteoclasts that break down bone - this is important during bone growth and healing where the bone needs to be broken down before new bone can form. In this disorder, there is an imbalance in this process, leading to bones becoming thicker. Also, as the bone is not completely broken down, toxic materials build-up that affect the growth of bone cells, resulting in short stature and distinctive facial features including a large head with a small face and chin, and misshaped teeth. The thickened bone is also more brittle and susceptible to breaking with individuals suffering numerous fractures.

It is widely suspected that the revered French artist Henri de Toulouse-Lautrec, famous for his posters and prints of Parisian nightlife, inherited this disorder. Born to an aristocratic family, his parents Count Alphonse and Countess Adèle de Toulouse-Lautrec, who were of average height, were first cousins. Their relatedness was likely to have contributed to their son's condition and at least three of his cousins, themselves the progeny of parents who were cousins, appeared to have suffered from the same condition. Standing only 1.53 meters tall with short legs, Henri also had shortened fingers and dental issues and showed the typical facial features of this disorder that resulted in his speech impediment and drooling. The bone fragility associated with this disorder led to him suffering numerous fractures; the two broken legs he sustained in his early teens never properly healed, leaving him with a limp and a reliance on a walking cane for the rest of his life.

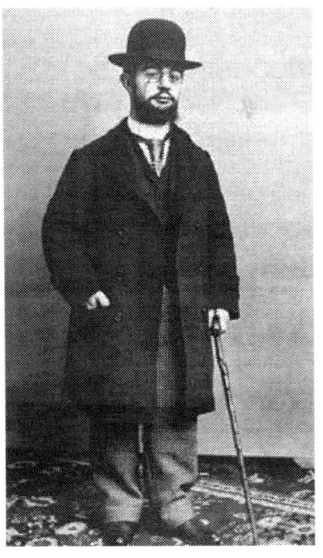

Henri de Toulouse-Lautrec, 1894

Another disorder associated with brittle bones is osteogenesis imperfecta (Gr. *osteo*, bone; *genesis*, formation, *imperfecta*, imperfect). Here various mutations in two genes for different types of collagen important for cartilage and bone lead to a spectrum of diseases ranging in severity from mild to lethal forms in early life. The Viking Ivar Ragnarsson, who invaded England in 865 AD, is thought to have suffered from one of the more severe types of this disease. He acquired the nickname *Ivar the Boneless* as he was supposedly unable to walk on his legs and so had to be carried around on a shield. The British actress, Julie

Fernandez, best known as *Brenda*, on the BBC comedy *The Office* also has a severe form of Osteogenesis Imperfecta. People with milder forms of the disease can appear relatively normal with average height and no defining characteristics other than an increased risk of broken bones. As such, this condition often goes undiagnosed. This has led to numerous instances of child abuse allegations due to increased bone fractures and breaks. In one of many similar examples in the UK, in 2011 two children were taken into care after social workers mistook the occurrence of eight fractures in the arms and legs in the youngest child just weeks after his birth, as evidence of abuse. It took 18 months for the services to realise the boy had been born with this condition and finally allow him to be reunited with his parents.

Some genetic syndromes result from developmental defects in early skeletal organisation. Mutations in genes involved in bone and joint formation in the spine or the process of separating vertebrae from one another during early development, lead to autosomal dominant or recessively inherited patterns of the disorder Klippel-Feil syndrome. This is characterised at birth by the abnormal joining of two or more vertebrae of the neck. This fusion leads to the appearance of a short neck that has restricted mobility. The English cricketer Gladstone Small was born with this disorder. He is most widely remembered for his bowling exploits that helped England retain the Ashes on Australian soil in the 1986-87 series.

There are a number of genetic disorders characterised by an altered arrangement of bone overgrowth where bone grows in the wrong place. Sclerosteosis and, its milder form, van Buchem disease result from increased activity of osteoblasts, the cells responsible for bone formation. A mutation disrupts the function of a protein whose normal job is to inhibit these osteoblasts and so control bone formation. This leads to progressive bone and

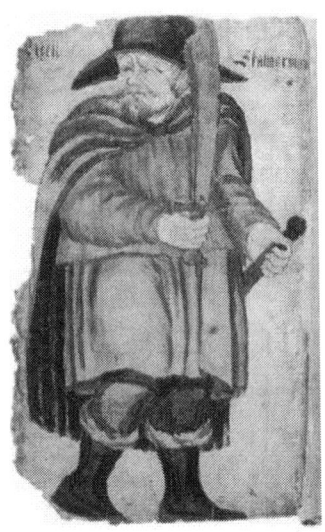

Egill Skallagrímsson, from a 17 century Icelandic manuscript

skeletal overgrowth, especially in the skull. Sufferers of these rare autosomal recessive disorders, though generally appearing normal at birth, later develop enlargement of the lower jaw, deafness and facial paralysis in childhood that can lead to life-threatening complications if the overgrowing skull compresses the brain. It has been suggested that the revered tenth-century Viking poet, Egill Skallagrímsson, may have suffered from this disease. Descriptions in medieval Icelandic narratives, known as Sagas, describe unusual disfigurements of his skull – *"a skull that could resist blows from an axe"* - and facial features. He also became deaf, often lost his balance, went blind, and suffered terrible headaches. The texts describe a similar characteristic skull deformation in his father, though not his brother, suggesting that the family may have carried the gene for this disorder, perhaps inherited in a dominant pattern.

Craniodiaphyseal dysplasia (*cranio*, cranium; *diaphysis*, the shaft of a long bone) is a rare autosomal recessive disorder that results in abnormal bone shape due to excessive deposition of calcium causing new bone to form. This can be particularly evident in the

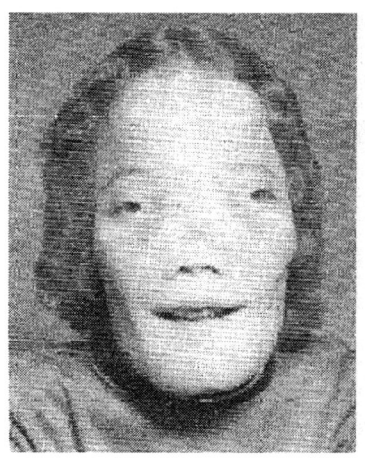

Rocky Dennis' junior high school yearbook photo, 1977

skull resulting in facial disfigurement. There is also narrowing of the holes within the skull, known as foramina, through which nerves and arteries pass through. This results in blindness, deafness, facial palsy and paralysis with most sufferers dying in childhood. This disorder is depicted in the 1985 biographical movie *The Mask* relating the life and early death of Roy L. "Rocky" Dennis, who suffered from this disease and died in 1980 at the age of 16.

*These things are good*

*Ice cream and cake*

*A ride on a Harley*

*Seeing monkeys in the trees*

*The rain on my tongue*

*And the sun shining on my face*


*These things are a drag*

*Dust in my hair*

*Holes in my shoes*

*No money in my pocket*

*And the sun shining on my face*

By Rocky Dennis (1961-1978)

In another example of uncontrolled bone growth, the body grows new bone at sites of an injury; fibrous tissues such as muscles, ligaments and tendons become replaced by bone. This occurs due to a mutation in a gene coding for a protein that becomes abnormally active, instructing connective tissues to repair by replacing with bone rather than their respective connective tissues. Known as fibrodysplasia ossificans progressiva (fibro; fibrous connective tissue, ossification; the process of bone formation, progressive) an individual's connective tissues slowly turn to bone. Autosomal dominantly inherited, this disorder affects around 1 person in every 2 million. One well-known sufferer was the American Harry Raymond Eastlack. Born in 1933, he started developing painful nodules in the neck and shoulders at the age of 10 years. This slowly progressed and towards the end

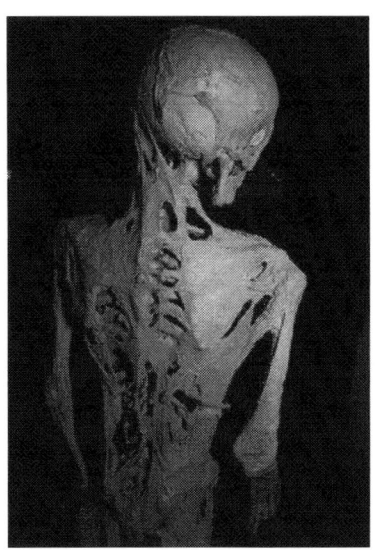

Skeleton of Harry Eastlack, in the Mütter museum in Philadelphia.

of his life, he was able only to move his lips. Before dying of pneumonia at the age of 39, he requested that his body be donated to science: his skeleton, pictured, is still on display at the Mutter Museum in Philadelphia showing how the muscles of his back had turned into sheets of bone.

There are a number of disorders that lead to individuals being born with extra bones or missing certain bones. Polydactyly (Gr. *poly*, many; *dactyl*; digit) is a relatively common disorder present in around 1 in 1000 births in the UK though is more common in African-Americans, typically occurring as a sixth little pinkie finger. This is sometimes inherited in a dominant pattern where extra fingers or toes are passed from parents to their children. This defect can also be a characteristic of some disorders, such as Ellis-van-Creveld syndrome, but generally, this anomaly occurs in the absence of any other medical defects. Some genetically isolated populations show higher incidences of this. One extreme

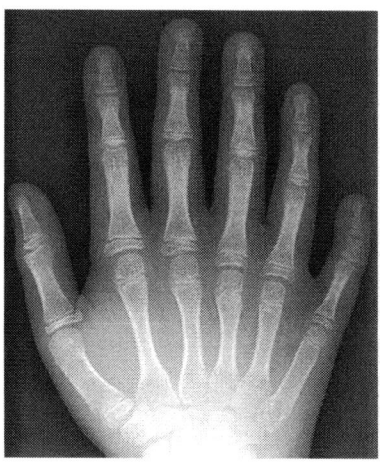

Polydactyly

example was seen in the inhabitants of the village of Eycaux in a remote mountainous region of France, who at the end of the last century nearly all presented with extra fingers and toes. This disorder can result from mutations in several different genes important in coordinating the patterning of limbs and digits as they develop in an unborn embryo to ensure we have the correct numbers of fingers and toes and that they grow in the right places.

Nowadays, these extra fingers or toes are often surgically removed during early life, such as in the case of the cricketer, Sir Garfield Sobers, the first player to hit six sixes in a single over of six consecutive balls in first-class cricket, or the *James Bond* actress Gemma Arterton of *Quantum of Solace*. However, there are people who keep their extra fingers and even put them to good use. Antonio Alfonseca has six fingers on each hand and six toes on each foot, a trait inherited through several generations of his family. Nicknamed *The Octopus*, he was a Major League Baseball pitcher for several clubs including the Chicago Cubs and Philadelphia Phillies in a career lasting a decade until 2007. People still argue over whether this allowed him to achieve extra and unusual forms of spin on a ball. A recent study has shown that people with extra fingers may have certain advantages, such as being able to type quicker and tie shoe-laces with a single hand, depending on how much dexterity the extra digit has. Legend has it that the renowned Italian composer and violinist Giuseppe Tartini had six fingers on his left hand that enabled him to play his famously complicated pieces, such as the *Devil's Trill Sonata*. However, extra fingers have certainly not been appreciated by all musicians. The American Blues guitarist and singer, Hound dog Taylor, cut off his extra sixth digit in a bar one night, shortly before he died of lung cancer, complaining that it had always hindered his guitar playing, getting caught between strings. Conversely, Django Reinhardt, arguably the greatest jazz guitarist of all time, with the use of only two fingers on his chord hand - after an accident removed the others - developed a characteristic style which has had such a lasting influence on many guitarists playing today. Tony Iommi from *Black Sabath* and Jerry Garcia from *The Grateful Dead* also played with missing fingers from the result of accidents

Polydactyly can also affect toes on either or both feet, often as an extra little toe as in the cases of film stars Drew Carey and Kate Hudson among many others who have decided not to have them surgically removed. Some forms of polydactyly present as an extra thumb. Often voted the sexiest, and one of the highest-paid Bollywood stars, Asian Hrithik Roshan, was born with an extra thumb fused to his other thumb one on his right hand. *"My thumb used to repel people in school. Today I am posting it to millions like you who I know are just like me. Beautifully imperfect,"* he has written. It is interesting to consider the numbers of models and actors and actresses famed for their attraction who likewise have imperfections.

In 2008, the American actor Ashton Kutcher showed the world he had webbed toes on live TV during the *Jonathan Ross Show*. Known as syndactyly (Gr. *Syn*; together), this can affect fingers or toes in which two or more digits fail to separate properly and appear to be stuck together. It results from a failure of programmed cell death that normally occurs between fingers and toes during foetal development. Affecting around 1 in 2000 births, it may also be familially inherited with different family members often showing variability

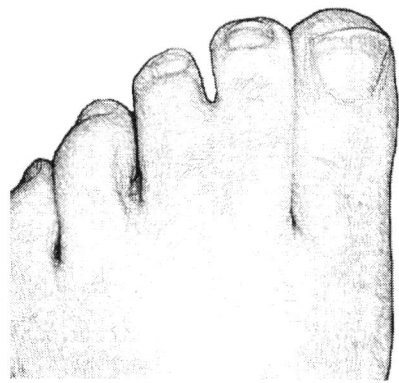

Syndactyly

with toes and fingers affected. In some Eastern cultures, this anomaly has been associated with divinity and wisdom; Buddha is said to have possessed webbed hands. But in Western cultures, such anomalies have tended to be viewed more negatively. However, the actions of the celebrities Ashton Kutcher and Rachel Stevens from *S Club 7* fame, who have both separately presented their webbed toes on live television, may have gone some way towards changing people's attitudes. Additionally, the American actress Danielle Panabaker famous for her roles in numerous *Disney* films and the Canadian actress and former model Tricia Helfer best known for the *Battlestar Galactica* series and *Lucifer* also both have syndactyl of the toes.

The model and wife of Justin Bieber, Hailey Bieber, has recently spoken out about a different digit defect complaining that people have been trolling her for her "crooked pinkie fingers". Known as Clinodactyly (Gr. *klínein*; to bend), a medical term describing a curved finger or toe, often the fifth finger, it is quite common and often passed through families in an autosomal dominant pattern.

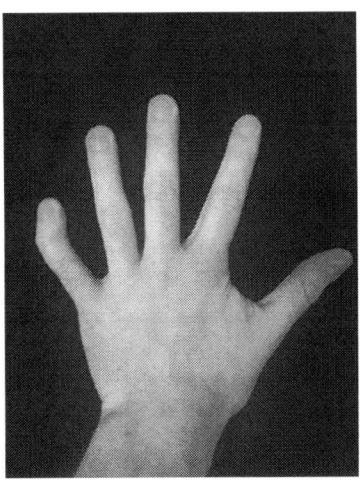

Clinodactyly

During the 2010 American Super Bowl, the American actress and model, Megan Fox appeared in a bubble bath for a raunchy mobile phone advert. However, for the close-up shots of her using the phone, the commercial organisers insisted on the use of a hand double. This is because she has a genetic condition called brachydactyly (Gr. *brachy*; short), describing the appearance of shortened thumbs. Often voted the most attractive woman

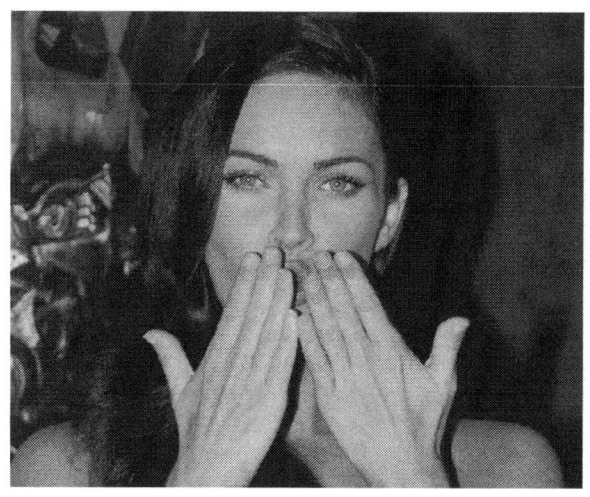

Megan Fox, 2009

alive she has also talked about being a victim of online trolls due to this small anomaly, or "beautiful imperfection" as Hrithik Roshan might describe it.

Other mutations can lead to the absence of one or more fingers or toes. Ectrodactyly (Gr. *Ektroma*; abortion/congenital absence), often known as cleft hand has been linked to a few genes that can result in autosomal dominant or X-linked recessive inheritance affecting either one or both hands. The Soviet chess Grandmaster, Mikhail Tal had ectrodactyly in his right hand. He was also an accomplished pianist. Feet may also be affected by the absence of toes. Early explorers to Zimbabwe returned with tales of "*ostrich-footed people*" due to individuals within a tribe born missing their three middle toes. And indeed, there are several communities in remote regions of the Kalahari Desert who have this disorder, exemplifying again the effects of inbreeding in isolated populations. Further individuals are born with affected hands and feet as seen in split-hand/split-foot malformation, caused by mutations in genes important in controlling growth and patterning of the developing limb. In the US there is the story of Grady Stiles, known in the circus as the *Lobster Man*, who had the condition passed on to him through four generations

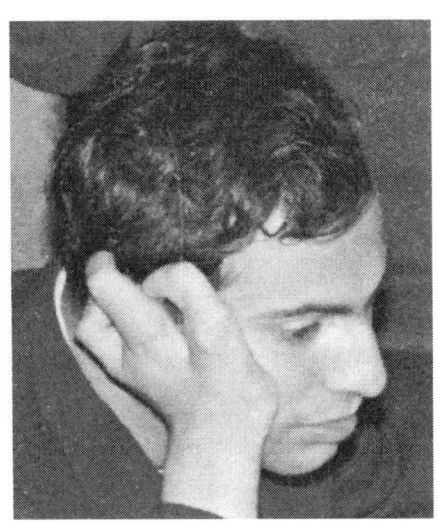

Mikhail Tal, 1961

of his family in a dominantly inherited manner. He, in turn, fathered four children, two of whom also had split hands and feet. While the Stiles family toured for years with a carnival, Grady, who was an alcoholic, would terrorise and beat his family. This culminated on one occasion when he went as far as to shoot and kill his daughter's fiancé on the eve of their wedding. Somehow, he managed to escape legal justice by playing on his deformity though he was not able to avoid the retribution of his wife who persuaded a neighbour, to murder him four years later in 1992.

British tennis star Fran Jones was born in 2000 with ectrodactyly. Following numerous operations in childhood, she has three fingers and a thumb on each hand, four toes on her left foot, and three toes on her right foot. Her missing digits means she holds her racket differently and has had to adapt her balance on her feet. Becoming one of the youngest players in the UK top 25, as of 2019 she is ranked in the top 300 in the world.

Mutations in other genes affecting the developing limb can lead to more severe phenotypes such as acheiropodia (Gr. *a*; absence, *cheiros*; hand, *podus*; foot) characterised by limbs, either arms or legs, that terminate in stumps missing hands or feet. This very rare condition can be caused by mutations in a gene important in limb development. Carl Hermann Unthan, known as the *Armless Fiddler*, was born in Prussia in 1848 missing arms and hands. From a young age, his father pushed him to do things for himself resulting in his ability to use his feet to grasp things and perform tasks that most people required their hands for, such as writing and even playing the violin. He toured America performing and, during the First World War, travelled around war hospitals giving motivational speeches to German amputees. His autobiography, written on a typewriter using his toes, and entitled *The Pediscript*, was published just after he died at the age of 80. Another sufferer of this was the French painter, Louis Ducornet, who as well as lacking arms, was also born with ectrodactyly of the feet, which he used to great effect in holding a paintbrush. One of his

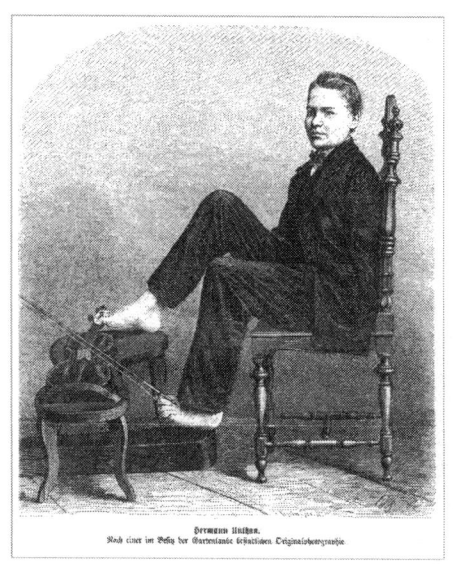

Carl Hermann Unthan, 1868

most famous pieces, the eleven-foot high depiction of *Mary Magdalene at the feet of Christ*, painted in 1840, still resides in his home town of Lille after it was purchased by the government.

Some birth defects occur where a bone or part of a bone in the leg or arm is missing. Fibular hemimelia is a very rare disorder, occurring in only 1 in 50,000 births in which a part or all of the fibular bone is missing. Most cases are sporadic though a small number of cases show an autosomal dominant pattern of inheritance with genes involved in the early development of the limb. A number of well-known Paralympians were born with this disorder and had their legs amputated at the knees, including the swimmer Jessica Long, and sprinters Liam Malone, Oscar Pistorius and Aimee Mullins who is now an actress and model.

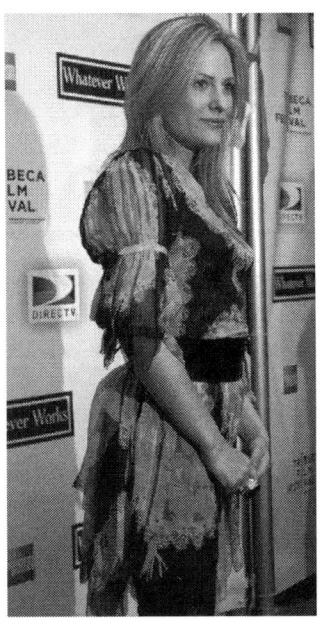

Aimee Mullins, 2009

One of the most common birth defects related to arms or legs, affecting around 1 in 1,000 new-borns in the UK, is clubfoot, also known as talipes. This results in one or both feet pointing downwards and inwards. Although exact mechanisms are still unknown, some genes have been identified as playing a major role and it can be passed down through families. Though this disorder can lead to a limp, the condition can usually be corrected in early childhood without any lasting problems. Indeed, the condition seems to have had little effect on the footballing career of the American Mia Hamm who won Gold in women's soccer in 1996 and has the accolade of having scored more international goals than any other player male or female. Arguably one of the most talented footballers who ever lived, the Brazilian, Garrincha, was born with very disfigured legs; a right leg bent inwards and a left leg also bowed and 6cm shorter. The American football stars Dan Marino, Troy Aikman, Charles Woodson and LeRoy Butler were all born with club feet. LeRoy's clubfeet were so bad that doctors had to break his legs and reset them while he was a toddler, forcing him to wear bulky braces on both legs until eight years old; 15 years later he would be named in the NFL 1990's All-Decade team. There are certainly many similar stories. The American figure skater, Kristi Yamaguchi, won Olympic gold for figure skating in 1992, only taking up the sport in childhood as therapy for her club feet. Tom Dempsey, born missing all his toes on his right foot and fingers on his right hand, in 1970 kicked the longest field goal in American football history, using his right foot - a record that has stood for 43 years.

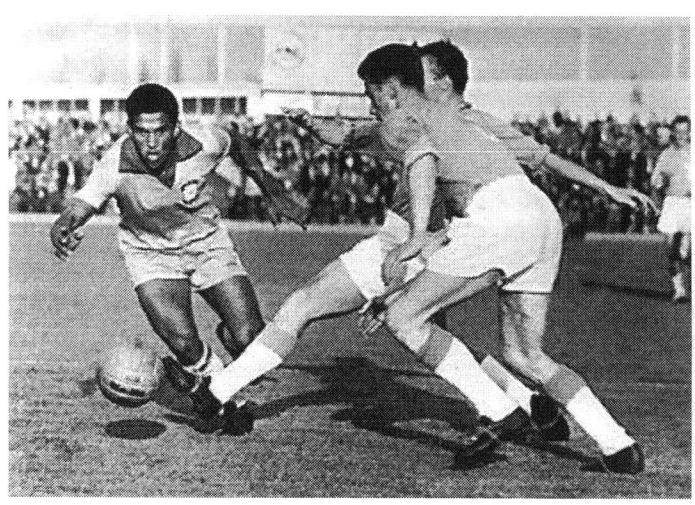

Garrincha playing for Brazil at 1962 World Cup

Two other common birth disorders are cleft lip and cleft palate that occur in around 1 in 700 births in the UK. Cleft lips appear as a gap or dent in the lip which can continue into the nose. Easily treated with surgery, this can result in a small scar that can be seen on the faces of actors including Stacy Keach of *Natural Born Killers*, Cheech Marin of *From Dusk Till Dawn* and British actor Tom Burke who starred in the BBC series *The Musketeers, War & Peace* and as the title character in *Strike*. Joaquin Phoenix, also has the characteristic scar reportedly from a microform cleft, describing a minor cleft that requires no surgery.

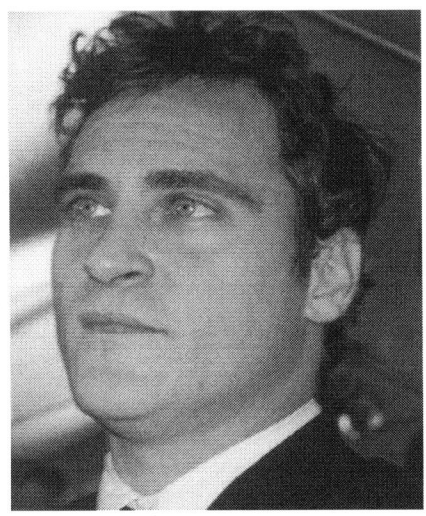

Joaquin Phoenix, 2005

A cleft palate is an opening, or split, in the roof of the mouth that occurs when the two plates of the skull that form the palate, i.e. the roof of the mouth, do not join together during the development of the foetus. Again, this is usually easily treated with surgery. Though generally not showing clear patterns of inheritance, there are genes involved in the development of cleft palates with affected parents having around 5 per cent increased risks of producing a child with the condition. In a similar way to cleft lips in actors, cleft palates have also had little effect on the voices of a number of well-known singers born with the condition and who had surgery. Examples include Richard Hawley, Canadian country and folk singer Rita MacNeil and Carmit Bachar, singer of the *Pussycat Dolls*, who has started up an organisation for children born with a cleft lip/palate called *Smile With Me*.

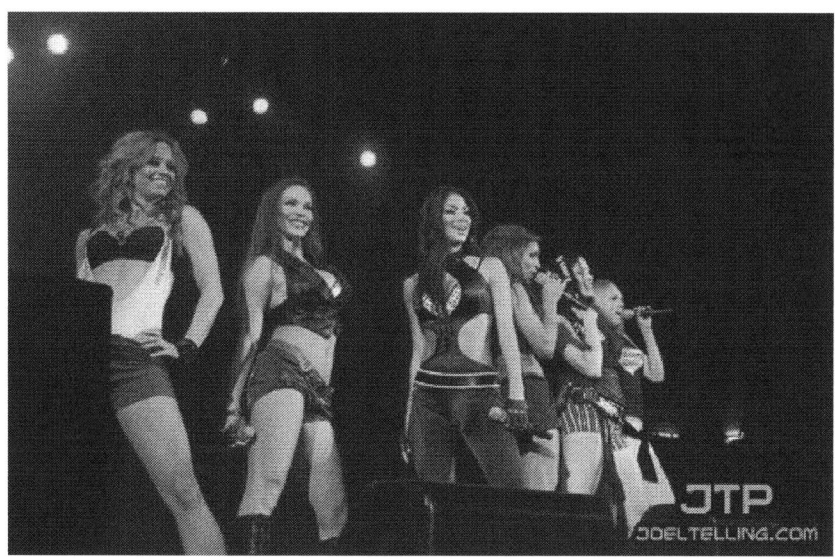

The Pussycat Dolls. Carmit Bachar, 2nd from the right. 2006

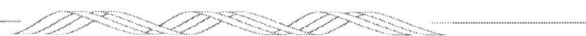

# CONNECTIVE TISSUE DISORDERS

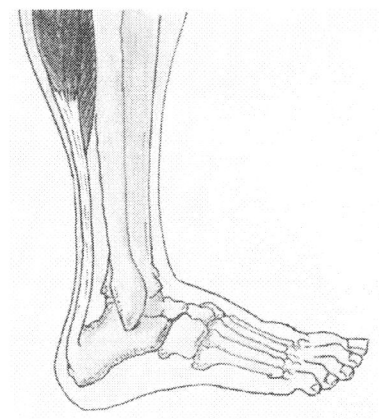

*I am not handsome, but when women hear me play, they come crawling to my feet.*

Niccolò Paganini

Our connective tissues surround and support the cells found within organs and other tissues. These include types of fibrous tissues consisting of various types of cells together with interlacing filaments of proteins such as collagens, elastin and fibrillin. Bone, ligaments, tendons and cartilage can also be thought of as more specialised forms of connective tissues. There are more than 200 heritable disorders of connective tissue resulting from defects in genes that are responsible for building these tissues. These can lead to disorders affecting skin, bones, joints, heart, blood vessels, lungs, eyes, and ears.

Collagen (Gr. *kola*; glue, *-gen*; making, referring to the ancient process of boiling animal bones for glue) is the main component of connective tissues, bone and cartilage. It is also responsible for providing strength and elasticity to connective tissues forming organ walls, blood vessels and the skin. Collagen is the most abundant protein in our body, making up around a third of all our total protein. There are several different types of collagen important for its different roles and these are produced by different genes. Mutations in these genes coding for collagens specific to different tissues lead to various diseases. For example, defects in collagens in skin and joints - different from those types important for bone in the previously mentioned osteogenesis imperfecta - result in a group of disorders named Ehlers-Danlos syndrome. This results in extremely loose joints and skin; large and small joints from knees and elbows to fingers can be excessively loose and can hyperextend and often dislocate while the skin can also be hyper-elastic, stretching beyond normal levels. The thin, translucent skin can also easily bruise and tear forming characteristic "cigarette paper" scars. In addition, there can be defects in the connective tissues of the intestines and arteries, that also need collagen to function, leading to heart and intestinal problems. Usually autosomal dominantly inherited, this disorder affects around 1 in 5,000 individuals, with the severity, characteristics and inheritance pattern dependent upon which disrupted collagen gene is inherited. Named after the two doctors who first detailed the features in 1900, the excessively flexible joints and characteristic scars were first described in the medical writings of Hippocrates, dating back to 400 BC.

Niccolò Paganini, proclaimed by many as the greatest violinist who ever lived, is suggested to have suffered from Ehlers-Danlos syndrome. He had bony hands, thin, almost translucent skin, large feet and an abnormally long neck. However, his hyperextensible

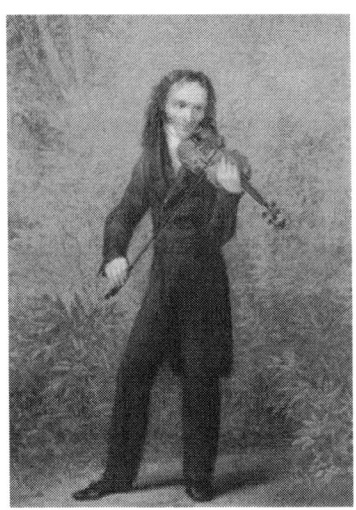

Niccolò Paganini by Georg Friedrich Kersting. 1830

joints allowed him incredible flexibility and many doubt he could have been so proficient without the abnormal dexterity in his fingers. So difficult was the music he wrote, that it was commonly thought that he had entered into a pact with the Devil. During his performances, he would often contort his body into seemingly impossible positions to play these pieces. However, his disease also led to numerous recurrent bouts of severe abdominal pain, which would trouble him for weeks to months at a time and leave him weak. In 1840, aged 57, Paganini died from internal haemorrhaging which is common among individuals with this disease. Incredibly, his widely rumoured association with the devil, meant that he was refused the Last Rites and his body was denied a Catholic burial. His son, who did not appear to have inherited his father's condition, desperately tried to find a cemetery who would take him. It would be fifty years, having been transported around Europe and stored in various cellars and temporary graves, before he was finally laid to rest in a fittingly grand tomb in La Villetta Cemetery in Parma.

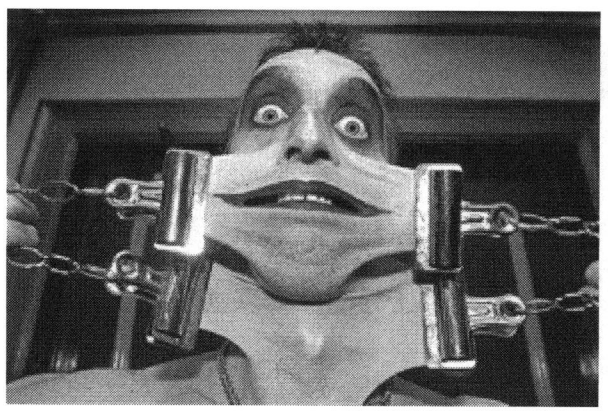

Gary "*stretch*" Turner, 2013

There have been many other performers with traits of Ehlers-Danlos syndrome who have made a living displaying their bendy bodies and stretchy skin. Some achieved celebrity status, with stage names such as *The India Rubber Man*, *The Elastic Lady*, and *The Human Pretzel*. Garry "*Stretch*" Turner, a pub landlord from Lincolnshire with this condition, holds the record for having the most clothes pegs attached to a face – 153! There are many other well-known people who have discussed their hyper-extendible joints associated with this disorder; British comedian and presenter Russel Kane has tweeted about the condition, while British singer and model Myleen Klass, revealed she was diagnosed aged 10 with the condition and showed off her double-jointed arms on *Celebrity Juice* in 2013.

Marfan syndrome is an autosomal dominant disorder affecting around 1 in 3,000 in the UK. It results from inheriting a mutation in a gene coding for a protein called Fibrillin, important in allowing tissues to stretch repeatedly without weakening. This produces a defective protein that is less able to keep connective tissue growth and elasticity in check leading to individuals growing tall with excessively long arms and legs and often long narrow faces. There are also serious complications involving the heart and major blood vessels that need Fibrillin to maintain strength during repeated contractions.

As this disorder associates with increased height together with long arms and legs, many sufferers become involved in sports associated with tall statures such as basketball and volleyball. However, the associated heart weaknesses, especially the aortic valve, can prove fatal especially during physical activity if not properly checked for. Flo Hyman, captain of the 1984 U.S. Olympic volleyball team and considered the best female volleyball player in the world, collapsed and died shortly after a game, with a subsequent autopsy revealing that

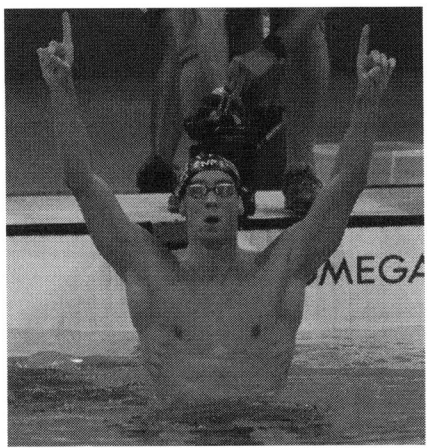

Michael Phelps, 2016

she had Marfan syndrome. There are a number of other well-known basketball and volleyball players who have died from heart attacks with suspected links to Marfan syndrome. In 2014, the National Basketball Association finally established a screening program of new players, prohibiting those with the disease and the associated heart defect from playing. Michael Phelps in his biography commented on his height, long hands and feet, and that if he reached out with his arms to form a "T" then his wingspan was "*very close*" to the length of his height; a wingspan longer than the height is a characteristic of the disease. Following doctors' advice for possible Marfan's complications, he has an electrocardiogram to test his heart for the typical weakness once a year which currently shows his aorta to be in good shape.

Another characteristic sign of Marfan syndrome is disproportionately long fingers and toes; a condition known as arachnodactyly, (Gr. *arachno*; spider). Sergei Rachmaninov, who is widely suspected to have had Marfan Syndrome, is said to have had one of the widest hand-spans of any pianist. He was able to cover a twelfth with his left hand – a span of approximately 12 inches from his little finger to his thumb. This disorder has also been linked to Charles de Gaulle and Osama bin Laden. Unusually tall for his family with a

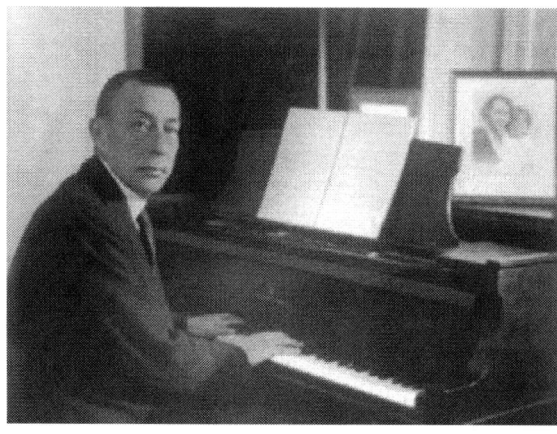

Sergei Rachmaninov, 1936

curved spine and narrow face Osama bin Laden was also reported to have had heart problems. Spanish actor Javier Botet, standing 6ft 6in (191 cm) tall has starred in some of Hollywood's biggest horror and fantasy productions. His tall, thin frame and flexibility, resultant of this disorder has led to him becoming one of the best "creature actors" in the industry with roles in a number of horror movies and an episode of *Game of Thrones*.

Another genetic disorder, in which individuals share a similar appearance to

Marfan's syndrome, is multiple endocrine neoplasia type 2b. This rare disorder results from mutations in a gene that leads to multiple cancers of endocrine glands, particularly the thyroid as well as Marfan features of lengthened limbs and long face and bumpy lips. It has been proposed that Abraham Lincoln may have inherited this due to his body shape and facial features. His progressive emaciation towards the end of his life, before he was shot, might have reflected cancer. There are suggestions that his sons Eddie, Willie, and Tad who died in childhood, and Abraham's mother might have also inherited this autosomal dominant disorder.

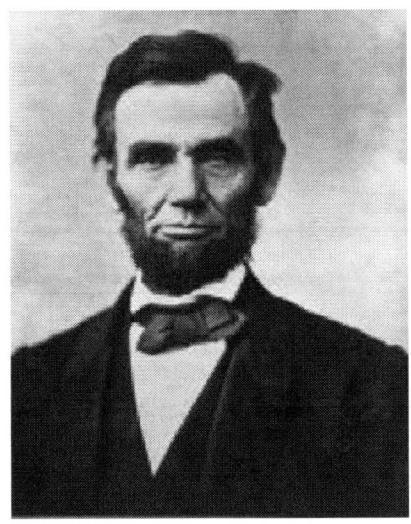

Abraham Lincoln, 1863

Elastin, as the name suggests, has a major elastic role in connective tissue allowing various tissues to resume its shape after stretching. Mutations disrupting this underlies the disorder cutis laxa (Lat. *cutis*, skin; *laxa*, loose), characterised by extremely loose skin. This group of rare autosomal dominant, recessive and X-linked disorders are characterised by skin that is inelastic and so hangs loosely in folds. Zara Hartshorn, from South Yorkshire, England, in 2016 had a face-lift at 16 years of age due to this rare condition that also affected her mother. Even while at school, she would often be mistaken for a woman in her forties until the operation that shaved years off the age of her appearance. In addition to the skin, other parts of the body, including the heart, blood vessels, joints, intestines, and lungs can also be affected. Now in her twenties, Zara raises important awareness of this condition.

Many other connective tissue disorders exist, particularly in association with autoimmune diseases. Scleroderma, for example, results from the immune system attacking the connective tissue under the skin resulting in scar tissue caused by the increased production of collagen leading to hard, thickened areas of skin. This can also sometimes affect internal organs and blood vessels. Although no specific genes are thought to cause scleroderma, certain variations in genes can increase a person's risk. These include human leukocyte antigen (HLA) complex genes that help the immune system distinguish the body's own proteins from foreign proteins, such as those produced by bacteria and viruses.

At the age of 56, the Swiss artist Paul Klee started to suffer from scleroderma, with fatigue, skin rashes, difficulty in swallowing, shortness of breath and pain in the joints of his

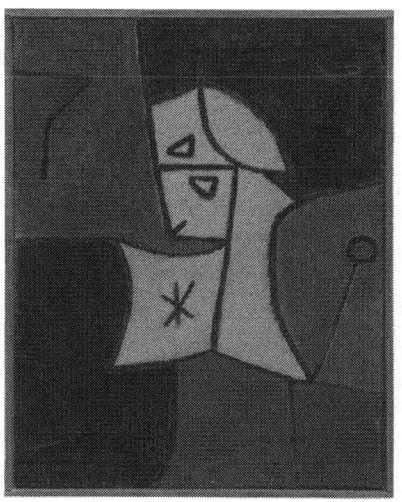

*Hoher wächter*, Paul Klee, 1940

91

hands and fingers that became so affected that he could barely hold a paint-brush. As a consequence, his artistic style drastically changed becoming simpler and less colourful, dominated by thick black lines; paintings for which he is perhaps most remembered.

# MUSCULAR DISORDERS

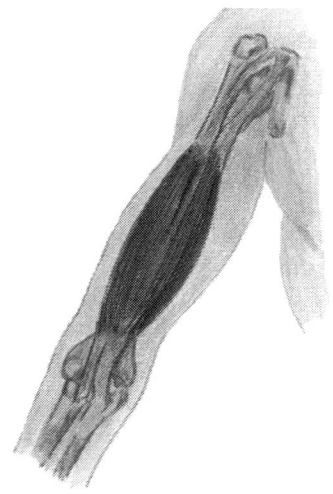

*I don't have much positive to say about motor neuron disease, but it taught me not to pity myself because others were worse off, and to get on with what I still could do. I'm happier now than before I developed the condition.*

Stephen Hawking

We have three main types of muscle. Skeletal muscle, which is anchored by tendons to the bone, is consciously used to move various parts of our bodies. Involuntarily muscle, also known as smooth muscle, moves without any conscious thought, such as in our intestines. Finally, there is the cardiac muscle responsible for keeping our hearts beating.

Inherited muscle diseases, known as muscle myopathies (Gr. *myo*; muscle), can occur through different mechanisms. Gene mutations can disrupt the function of important proteins needed for muscle cell growth or in in important proteins regulating electrical impulses needed to move muscles and the nerve cells connecting to muscles. Mutations can also affect mitochondrial important in providing the high levels of energy that muscles need. In contrast, some genes can result in increased muscle growth and function.

The most common inherited forms of progressive muscle weakness and wasting symptoms are Duchenne muscular dystrophy and Becker muscular dystrophy (Gr. *dys*; bad, *–trophy*; nourishment/development). X-linked recessively inherited, both diseases result from mutations in the same gene on the X chromosome that produces a protein important in strengthening muscle fibres. As this is X-linked recessive, the two disorders predominantly affect boys. The more severe Duchenne, that affects around 1 in every 3,500 males born, results from mutations that prevent any functional protein from being produced, while the milder Becker mutations still allow for this protein to retain some function. Consequently, Becker results in relatively milder effects and a later age of onset with patients surviving into their 40s. Symptoms for Duchenne, however, start earlier around 3-7 years old with difficulties in standing up and walking which worsens with most individuals confined to a wheelchair by age 12 and dying of respiratory complications by their 20s.

Alfredo, known as *Dino*, Ferrari was born in 1932 and suffered from muscular dystrophy. Though leaving him very weak, he continued to work with his father Enzo at his

94

Ferrari car manufacturing company on the development of a 1.5 L DOHC V6 engine for F2, which was later renamed in his honour when he passed away at the age of 24 years old. After his death, his distraught father, who wore black sunglasses every day for the rest of his life, founded the Dino Ferrari Foundation in Milan, which is still one of the most important research centres in the world for muscular dystrophies.

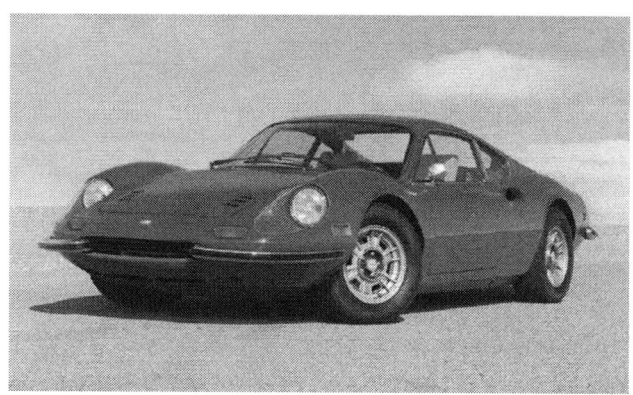

1972 Ferrari Dino 246GT

In 1876 a Danish physician, Dr Julius Thomsen, wrote a paper on an inherited painless muscle stiffness in his limbs and, typically, an inability to release his handgrip rapidly. He described how he could trace back the condition to his maternal great-grandmother born in 1742. Supposedly highly sensitive about his familial condition, he was simply trying to provide a medical explanation to support the exemption from military service of the youngest of his three affected sons. This was the first documented account of a myotonic disorder (Gr. *myo*, muscle; *tonic*, strength), characterised by muscles that can contract normally but have decreasing power to relax. These diseases result from a block in the flow of electrical impulses across the muscle cell membrane; without the proper flow of charged particles, the muscle cannot return to its relaxed state after it has contracted. Generally, this results in painless muscle stiffness in the limbs and an inability to release the handgrip rapidly. There is usually have no effect on a person's lifespan. One form, known as Thomsen's myotonia congenita, named after Julius Thomsen, is caused by inheriting a mutation in a gene affecting the function of a chloride channel. This regulates the flow of chloride ions across a cell membrane during the generation of an electrical impulse that is an important step in the contraction of muscle cells. There is a breed of domestic goat with mutations in a similar gene, known as the fainting goat. Their muscles freeze for roughly 10 seconds when the goat is startled and tries to suddenly move, causing the animal to collapse on its side. These have been used to protect prized sheep from wolf attacks, the idea being that these poor animals are dined upon first.

There are other ion channels that play a role in initiating muscular contractions when stimulated by nerves. Hypokalemic periodic paralysis (*Hypo*, less; *kalemic*, calcium) is a disorder resulting from mutations to a gene coding for an ion channel that mediates the influx of calcium into and out of cells. Affecting around 1 in 100,000 individuals this autosomal dominant inherited condition results in intermittent episodes of muscle weakness and sometimes paralysis, usually lasting less than a day, where muscle reflexes decrease and

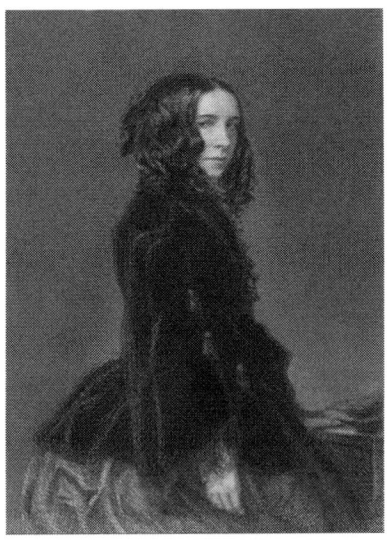

Elizabeth Barret Browning by Thomas Oldam Barlow

go limp, particularly in the shoulders and hips. This is often induced by strenuous exercise and foods with high levels of salt or sudden changes in temperature. The English poet Elizabeth Barrett Browning (1806–1861) is thought to have suffered from this disease describing in a diary her overwhelming weakness after fasting or exercise "*Very unwell – could scarcely get down stairs, my legs trembled so much.*" This may have led to her self-prescribing opiates from an early age with suggestions that this may have greatly influenced her style of writing.

Myotonic dystrophy, of which there are two types is characterised by wasting and weakness of muscles in the arms and legs. This autosomal dominant disorder, that affects around 1 in 30,000, is caused by mutations in either of 2 genes that produce proteins that play a role in communication within cells important for the correct functioning of cells in the heart and skeletal muscles. Generally developing in adulthood, this also leads to prolonged muscle contractions, together with slurred speech, temporary locking of the jaw and a mask-like expression, typically with drooping eye-lids, known as ptosis (Gr. *pto-* to fall). However, symptoms can vary considerably together with life expectancy depending on the severity of breathing and heart problems.

It has been suggested that the pharaoh Akhenaton, of the Eighteenth dynasty of Egypt, might have had myotonic dystrophy judging only from artistic representations of him. Reigning from around 1350 BC he is portrayed with a strikingly bizarre appearance - a long face, thin and hollow cheeks, a half-open mouth and the characteristic drooping eyelids. The revered Greek military commander Alexander Ypsilantis (1792-1828) may have also suffered from this disorder with portraits showing ptosis, and weakness of the face muscles. His younger brother Demetrius, who also fought with him in the Greek war of independence against the Ottoman Empire, also appears to have suffered from the ailment in addition to other ancestors of his.

Ptosis can affect one eye or both eyes and may be present at birth or acquired later in life. When present at birth, known as congenital ptosis there are often defects in muscle structure in the upper eyelid. There are many described cases of ptosis passed down

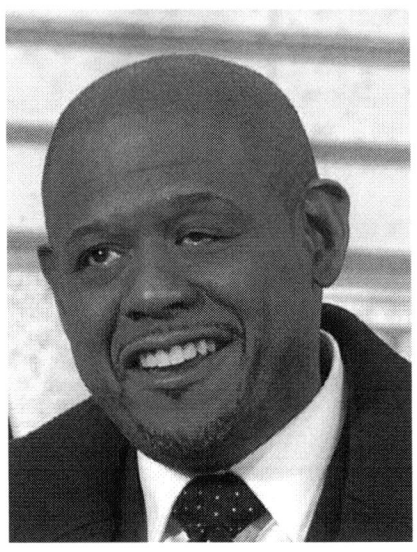

Forest Whitaker, 2009

through families suggesting there are some genes involved. The American actor, Forest Whitaker, suffers from a hereditary form of ptosis affecting his left eye, that also affected his father. Winning numerous awards including an Academy Award for best actor for his portrayal of Idi Amin in *The Last King of Scotland*, critics often comment that the eye defect gives him an "*intriguing*" "*lazy, contemplative look*". He has mentioned considering having surgery to correct it, not for cosmetic reasons, but because it affects his vision when he looks up.

In 2019, English bodybuilder Eddie Hall, the winner of the 2017 World's Strongest Man Competition, announced that he has what's commonly referred to as the 'Hercules's

Gene'. He currently holds the world record for heaviest deadlift at 500 kgs (1,102 lbs). The gene mutation he has inherited allows the body to build more muscle mass. In contrast to gene defects leading to muscle loss or weakness, some genes, when altered, can lead to increased muscle strength and growth. Belgian Blue cattle contain a cow equivalent of this same mutant gene disrupting the protein, myostatin, whose normal role is to limit muscle growth. As a result, they produce a third more muscle than normal cows. This gene was first discovered by scientists in a particular strain of mutant mice, named *Mighty mice*, that had twice as much muscle as normal. It appears that dog breeders have been inadvertently selecting for this same gene for many years in whippet racing. A study showed that a high number of dogs in the top racing classes had one copy of this mutant gene. Dogs that inherit two copies of the mutant gene are extremely muscular and are known as bully

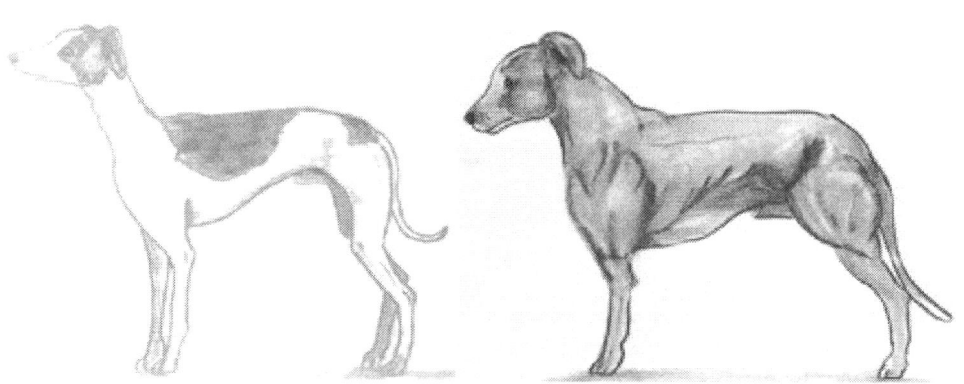

Whippet and a bully whippet

whippets. Contrary to the name and appearance, however, they have a very placid temperament but too much muscle for them to be as fast as those whippets inheriting only one mutant copy of this gene.

Liam Hoekstra, born in Michigan in 2005, was given up for adoption as an infant by his mother who was worried, he had a severe medical condition as he just seemed different. At the age of 5 months, he could walk upstairs upright and at 1 year old, he could do chin-ups. At the age of 3, doctors tested his strength, and found he was as strong as an average 7-year-old, with 40 per cent more muscle than others his age. When his blood and DNA was he was found to have a genetic deficiency in myostatin. Perhaps he is genetically programmed to grow up be a future World's Strongest Man?

In 2018 China's Ministry of Science and Technology announced it would scour athletes' blood for so-called 'Olympic genes', and that all Chinese athletes competing in the 2022 Winter Olympics would be selected after undergoing "*complete genome sequencing*" to test athletes for "*speed, endurance and explosive force*". There are dozens of genes believed to control up to half of our athletic ability and the idea that genetic testing can be used to predict a person's sporting talent before that person has even pulled on their sports shoes, is an old one. In 2005, a rugby team in Australia announced that it would start testing players for a gene called ACTN3 in an effort to predict an individual's sprinting speed. One wonders to what end future young athletes might be selected using their genetic sequences rather than their actual performances.

One of the most widely studied genes associated with athletic performance, ACTN3, is also known as the 'Sprinter's gene". It provides the instructions to produce a protein that helps fast-twitch muscles contract powerfully at high speeds. People who produce more of this protein are predisposed to be more adapted to sprinting instead of long-distance running. However, if you have a different variant of this gene, your fast-twitch muscle fibres will behave more like slow-twitch muscle fibres - some studies show this variant is more often found in endurance athletes. Importantly though, one more recent study looking at U.S. and Jamaican sprinters did not find higher numbers of the ACTN3 gene. It is therefore not entirely clear whether such an ACTN3 test might have found Usain

Bolt.

There are a number of other genes associated with muscle and athleticism and a number of companies that offer genetic tests on such genes to predict athletic performance. Another gene often discussed is the ACE gene which codes for the ACE protein that is

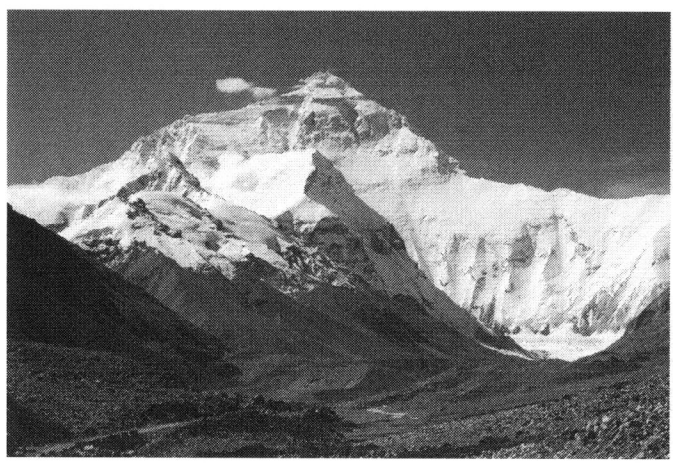

Mount Everest

important in regulating blood pressure and the balance of fluids and salts in the body. People have a different version of the gene either missing or containing in a tiny extra chunk of DNA that affects the ability of the genes to produce more or less ACE protein. Some studies have found that elite mountaineers and Sherpas tend to have a version of the gene missing the extra bit of DNA suggesting a beneficial physiological role in adapting to a high-altitudes.

Motor neurons connect the spinal cord and brain with muscle fibres to allow muscle contraction. For muscles to function, grow and survive they must be constantly stimulated by the motor neurons; if not, the muscles weaken and waste away. Diseases associated with the death of motor neurons lead to progressive paralysis of the body, often starting in the hands and feet and proceeding up the arm or leg, and also spasticity where muscles twitch, become tight and spasm.

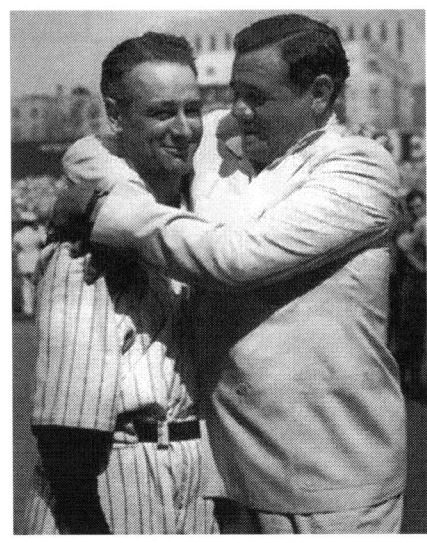

Lou Gehrig (left)and Babe Ruth at Yankee Stadium on July 4, 1939

On July 4, 1939, almost 62,000 people crowded into the Yankee Stadium to hail and applaud one of the true greats of baseball as he announced his retirement. *The New York Times* reported, "*perhaps as colourful and dramatic a pageant as ever was enacted on a baseball field*". Nicknamed '*the Iron Horse*' for his durability, he set the record for the most consecutive games played, 2,130 - a record that stood for 56 years. Eventually, he was forced to remove himself from the line-up - the manager refused to drop him - after he began to realise his performances on the field were becoming hampered by something he described as "*a cold in his back*". This might have been the first symptom of his debilitating disease. Retiring in 1939 at age 36, following his diagnosis, he told the crowd "*Fans, for the past two weeks, you've been reading about a bad break. Today I consider myself the luckiest man on the face of the earth. I have been in ballparks for 17 years and have never received anything but kindness and encouragement from you fans*". The Yankees retired his number, 4, making him the first player in Major League

Baseball to receive this accolade. Two years later he died. Forever referred to as Lou Gehrig's disease in the U.S., amyotrophic lateral sclerosis (Gr. *a*, absence; *myo*, muscle; *trophic*, nourishment) (ALS), also known as motor neuron disease, affects about 1 in 30,000 people. While most cases seem to appear at random, some inherited cases are the result of mutations in a gene important for clearing free radicals from cells. Different mutations in this gene affect the age symptoms begin and how fast the disease progresses: either rapid deterioration in later life or more gradual symptoms in early life. The great British actor, David Niven's symptoms appeared at the age of 70; he died just 3 years later. This was first noticed by the public when his slurring speech during an interview for the BBC in 1981 led

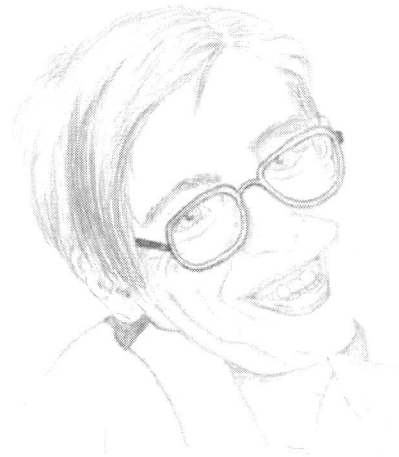

Stephen Hawking

many to wrongly assume he was drunk. Stephen Hawking, one of our greatest physicists in recent times, developed the disease at the young age of 21 and lived with the condition for 55 years. There also seem to be numerous environmental risk factors for developing amyloid lateral sclerosis. For example, a number of professional Italian soccer players have suffered leading people to suggest that heading footballs or pesticides on soccer fields may play some role. However a number of well-known sportspeople have suffered with the condition: Joost van der Westhuizen, widely considered one of South Africa's greatest rugby players died in 2017 from the condition, and Scottish rugby legend Doddie Weir announced he had been diagnosed with the disease in 2019.

Although ALS is the most well-known motor neuron disease, it is not the most common. Spinal muscular atrophy is 5-times more prevalent than ALS, though perhaps receives relatively less publicity as because most affected people tend to die very young. There are three main types of spinal muscular atrophy. The acute type usually results in death within the first year, while a less severe form presents between the ages of 5 and 15 years with a comparatively slower progression of weakness. However, as with most genetic diseases of this type, rate of progression of symptoms and life expectancy are variable with some sufferers surviving into adulthood. Ami Ankilewitz long outlived his predicted life expectancy. Working as a 3D animator in Israel, at age 36 he created and stared in an award-winning documentary, *39 Pounds of Love*, chronicling his pursuit of a lifelong ambition – an American road trip to find the doctor who predicted he would not live more than a few years.

The Australian actress Kate Hood, best known for her role on the television series *Prisoner*, started to developed weakness in her legs in her late 30s, falling over for no apparent reason. Known as hereditary spastic paraplegia this a group of inherited disorders characterised by progressive weakness, spasticity or stiffness of the legs that typically slowly progress so that individuals usually require the assistance of a cane or wheelchair. The genetics of this disorder are highly complicated with more than 80 genetic types of this disease currently described. Finally diagnosed in her mid-40s Kate Hood now uses a wheelchair full time and started a new career as a disabled actor, writer and commercial voice-over artist, winning awards for her audio book narrations.

# SKIN DISORDERS

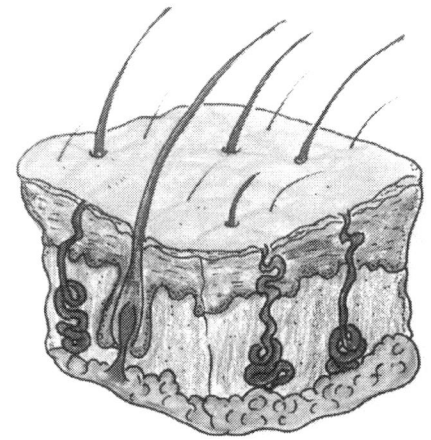

*High school was when I really learned about ignorance and prejudice and cruelty. Kids learn from society and parents.*

Michael Berryman

The skin is the largest organ in the body, both in weight and in surface area, and separates our body's internal environment from our external environment. It protects us from water loss and uses specialised pigment cells, called melanocytes, to protect us from ultraviolet radiation. Our skin contributes to the body's supply of vitamin D and helps regulate body temperature and metabolism. Skin is composed of an outermost epidermis (Gr. *epi*, on; *derma*, skin) followed by the dermis and then the subcutaneous layer containing fat cells. The epidermis is composed mainly of skin cells, known as keratinocytes, and melanocyte cells, while the dermis contains blood vessels, nerves, hair follicles, muscle, glands and lymphatic tissue. Each square cm of human skin can consist of up to four million cells, 24 hairs, 35 oil glands, 6.1 meters of blood vessels, 246 sweat glands, 7,480 sensory cells, 23,622 pigment cells, and more than 393 nerve endings.

Keratinocytes produce strong structural proteins called keratins (Gr. *keras*; horn). These proteins enable the cell to keep a robust rigid structure and they are also the main component of nails, hair, feathers and horns. There are over 30 different types of keratin proteins, important for their different roles in our bodies. Mutations in genes for keratin proteins or other genes important in the epidermis can lead to the skin either becoming too hard, as seen in various types of ichthyosis, or too delicate resulting in epidermolysis bullosa disorders. As the keratinocytes develop, they move up the skin layers producing different types of these keratin proteins forming rigid scaffolds in the cells. As the cells reach the layers of the stratum corneum they die forming the dead cell layer of our outermost skin. An increase in this process occurs in psoriasis.

Ichthyoses (Gr. *ichthys*; fish) results from an overproduction of skin keratin or loss of moisture leading to very thick and tough scaly skin that can sometimes resemble the scales of a fish. Ichthyosis vulgaris (Lat. vulgaris; common) is the most common form and is caused by mutations in a gene coding for a protein that normally binds to keratin and regulates the skin pH and retention of moisture. Loss of function of this protein in this disorder leads to hard dry scaly skin while other less damaging mutations in this same gene have been found in people with eczema. Many sufferers from this condition have often appeared as *Alligator* or *Lizard* people in various sideshows. One sufferer, Emmitt Bejano, known by his stage-name of *The Alligator-Skinned Man*, made the headlines when he eloped with Priscilla Lauther, another side-show performer known as *The Monkey Girl*, who suffered another disorder. Priscilla's foster father disapproved of Emmitt Bejano, and so when the two ran off together to marry in 1932, a local newspaper famously penned the headlined: *"Monkey Girl Kidnapped by Alligator Man."* They remained together until Emmitt Bejano died in 1995. They had only one child who died not long after birth.

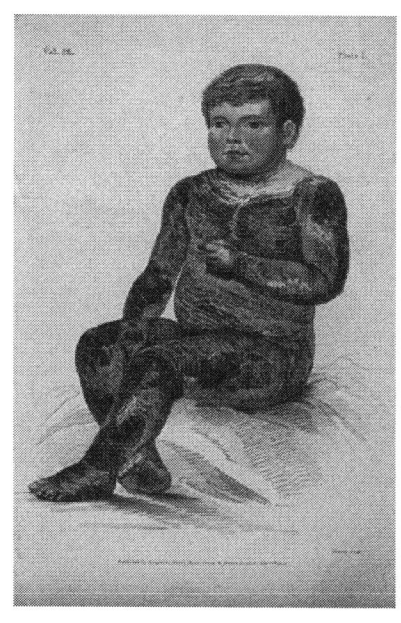

A boy with icthyosis by R.W. Sievier, 1818

There is a description of a man, Edward Lambert, born in Suffolk in 1717 who earned his living by appearing in travelling circuses under the name of *The Porcupine Man*. Born to unaffected parents, subsequent generations of his family, including several of his affected sons inherited the condition and carried on the family trade of exhibiting themselves around Europe. There is a type of related skin disorder called ichthyosis hystrix

(Gr. *hystrix*; porcupine) resulting in heavily uneven skin forming ridges and spikes that descriptions and a drawing of Edward Lambert might suggest he had. One of the most severe types of ichthyosis is lamellar ichthyosis (Gr. *Lamella*, thin plate) in which individuals have large, dark, plate-like scales covering their skin on most of their body. Affecting around 1 in 100,000, babies are born with a thick membrane which dries, cracks and peels off, leaving the baby with bright red underlying skin.

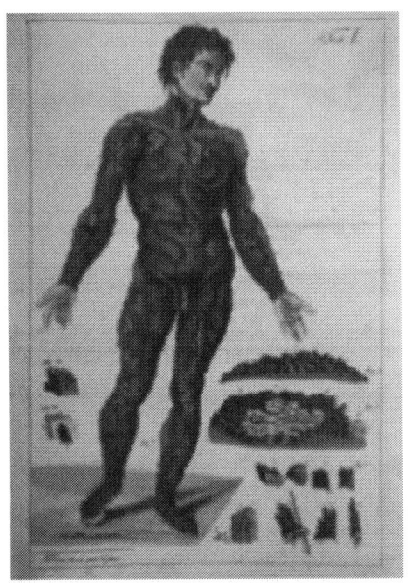

Edward Lambert

Mutations in other genes important in the epidermis can lead to severe skin fragility. Epidermolysis bullosa (Gr. *lysis*; release/loosening, Lat. *bulla*; bubble/blister) results in a person's skin being so fragile, that even clothing or warm temperature can lead to tearing or blistering. This autosomal dominant disease results from mutations that disrupt keratin proteins. Depending upon which keratin proteins are affected, skin fragility can vary from the mild epidermolysis bullosa simplex to the severe dystrophic epidermolysis bullosa. One sufferer of this disorder, Jonny Kennedy, was the subject of the film documentary *The Boy*

*Whose Skin Fell Off,* detailing the final months of his life. A scene shows his mother changing the protective bandages for his blisters that covered three-quarters of his body. As she does so, thick layers of his skin also tear off. A tireless campaigner for recognition of the disease, he died in 2003 from skin cancer, for which there is an increased risk with this disease.

The human skin generally sheds itself at a rate of about a million cells every 40 minutes, around three-quarters of a kilogram a year! This process accelerates in conditions of excessive keratinocyte proliferation such as in psoriasis (Gr. *psora*; itch), resulting from hyperactivity of the immune system. A number of different genes, which regulate the immune system, are suspected of causing the disease leading to an autoimmune reaction. A number of well-known singers and models have suffered from this. The singer and actress, LeAnn Rimes is a prominent spokesperson for *Stop Hiding from Psoriasis* a campaign that raises awareness for the disease whilst Cindi Lauper, is also a spokeswoman for the *National Psoriasis Foundation.* The supermodel Cara Delevingne has talked about suffering severe psoriasis flare-ups that were sometimes noticeable on the catwalk. Using thick layers of

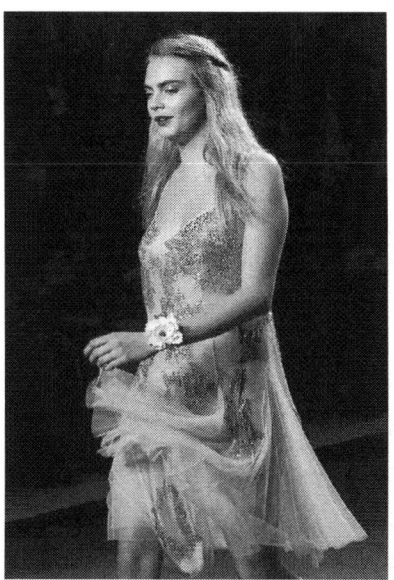

Cara Delevingne

make-up to cover it up, she has linked it to stress and commented that some people avoided touching her thinking it might be contagious. Kim Kardashian West has also been vocal about her psoriasis, that started to develop around the aged of 30, and has suggested she thinks that she inherited it from her mother. In *Keeping Up With the Kardashians* she said: "*There's nothing I can do about it, so there's no reason why I should feel uncomfortable.*" There are many other well-known models and celebrities that suffer from this condition.

The British author and playwright Dennis Potter suffered from a form of psoriasis known as psoriatic arthritis that, in addition to affecting the skin, also causes arthritis in the joints. This was diagnosed aged 26 and led to frequent hospitalisations. Often unable to move without great pain, sometimes he was so immobile that he could only write by strapping a pen to his hand – this is a famous scene he recreates in one of his most celebrated plays *The Singing Detective*. This condition also affects the US golfer Phil Mickelson. In 2010, pain in his ankles, fingers, and wrists left him bedridden with the pain. Amazingly, following treatment, he was able to continue playing, winning his third Masters later that year.

Skin develops from the ectoderm, the outer of the three primary germ layers in the very early developing embryo. Errors in this can lead to an absence of associated structures such as hair, nails, teeth and sweat glands. This occurs in the disorder, ectodermal dysplasia (Gr. *ecto*; outside, *derma*; skin, *dysplasia*), a group of diseases characterised by a lack of teeth, hair, sweat glands and nails. The most common form is X-linked hypohidrotic ectodermal dysplasia (Gr. *hypo*; reduced, *hidrotic*; sweating), caused by mutations in a gene on the X chromosome coding for a protein controlling development of the ectoderm. The American actor Michael Berryman was born with this disorder, his unusual appearance getting him roles in a number of horror movies. His first major film, *The Hills have Eyes* was shot in the

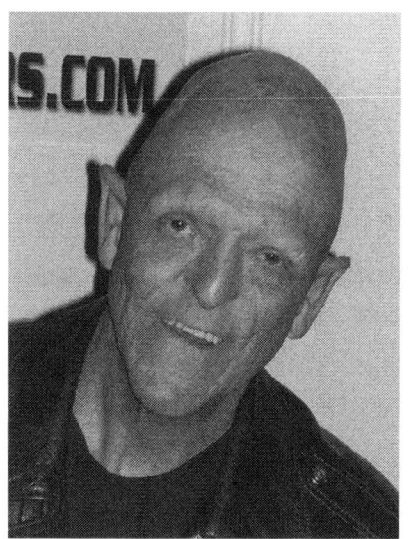

Michael Berryman

middle of the Nevada desert – surely the worst possible place to be for someone lacking sweat glands. He later described that he had to rest often to avoid overheating. There is a breed of bald, toothless dogs that contain defects in a similar gene. Known as the Mexican Hairless Dog, they were supposedly bred by the Aztecs as a type of bed warmer.

The skin contains millions of nerve endings that allow us to perceive sensations including pressure, temperature and pain. Some genetic conditions lead to the disruption or loss of these different neurons and can render an individual insensitive to these sensations. There is a hospital in Northern Sweden that, for many years, had been treating patients with broken bones who felt no pain. In the early 2000s, an orthopaedic surgeon, Jan Minde, when investigating the condition, found that many individuals suffered from a condition known as congenital insensitivity to pain. They all descended from a couple, Hindrich Kyro and his wife, who settled in the area in 1674 founding the town of Vittangi. Many were at increased risk of bone breakages as they were unable to protect themselves. One girl described how she enjoyed jumping on to floors and landing on her kneecaps as she liked the funny cracking sound they made. Swedish author, Steig Larsson's book *The Girl Who Played with Fire* described a tough villain as suffering from a similar disease, feeling no pain despite having nails driven through him. A related disorder, insensitivity to pain with anhidrosis (*Anhidrosis*, lack of sweat), leaves sufferers unable to feel pain or temperature. This results in an inability to control body temperature and sweating and many individuals injure themselves in ways that would normally be prevented by feeling pain and temperature. Even sitting or sleeping, in positions that would be considered uncomfortable to most, lead to damage of joints in these individuals. Many sufferers die young from overheating.

Neurofibromatoses are autosomal dominant disorders characterised by the development of a type of tumour, known as a neurofibroma, from the cells and tissues covering nerves. The two major types are neurofibromatosis type 1, in which tumours grow on or under the skin, and neurofibromatosis type 2 resulting in tumours within the brain. Both these result from mutations in genes that acts as a tumour suppressor, a term used for a gene that plays an important role in keeping cells from growing and dividing too rapidly or in an uncontrolled way. Mutations in such genes can lead to the production of a non-functional version of the protein that cannot regulate cell growth and division and so cause tumours.

In neurofibromatosis type 1, the first symptoms are usually flat and pigmented birthmarks known as café-au-lait spots that appear during childhood. Neurofibromas then develop over time, as well as skeletal problems and often small bumps on the iris, known as Lish nodules. The British actor, presenter and campaigner, Adam Pearson, was diagnosed with neurofibromatosis type 1 when he was five years old. Working on the Channel 4 documentary series *Beauty & The Beast: The Ugly Face of Prejudice* (2011), Adam Pearson has raised fantastic awareness of the condition. He has also worked as a reporter on TV's *Tricks of the Restaurant Trade* and BBC *One's The One Show*. Interestingly, he has a twin brother, with the same inherited gene and condition, but suffers only memory loss without any of the visible symptoms that Adam Pearson has, illustrating the variability in the symptoms of this disease between affected individuals. It has been suggested that the depiction of *Quasimodo* reflects Neurofibromatosis type 1, with a description of having cysts on his skin and lumps and bumps together with a curved spine and a large head. The renaissance painter Andrea

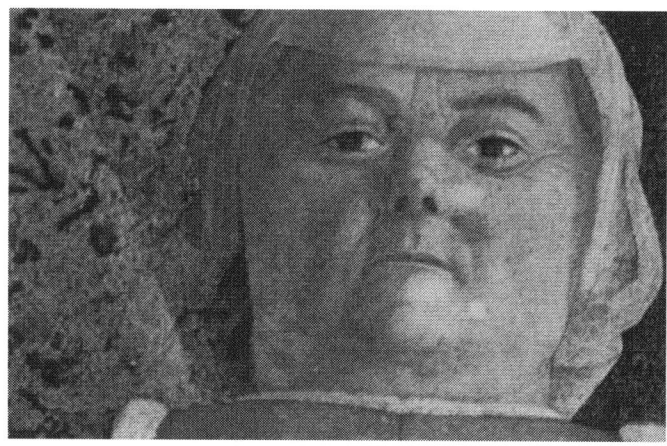

Andrea Mantegna, *Portrait of a maidservant affected by dwarfism*, ca 1470

Mantegna (1431–1506), as part of a series of frescoes in the *Bridal Chamber in the Gonzaga Palace in Mantua*, painted a servant with neurofibromas on the face and café au lait spots on the cheeks and one on the chin together with Lish nodules in both irises. Painted around 85 years before the first medical description in 1592 by the Italian naturalist Ulisse Aldrovrandi and 375 years before being officially recognised by the German pathologist Friedrich Daniel von Recklinghausen, it highlights the incredible clinical detail with which many artists have depicted subjects over the ages.

Twenty years earlier, before publishing the paper on neurofibromatosis in 1881 von

Recklinghausen, while working as an assistant to the famed Rudolf Virchow in the Institute for Pathological Anatomy in Berlin, presented a case of an infant who had died with several tumours in the heart and a large number of scleroses in the brain. These were almost certainly the characteristic tumours and brain growths of the disorder tuberous sclerosis (Tubor/root-like growths in the brain that become sclerotic, i.e. calcified and hardened). He actually failed to recognise this a distinct disease, and its name would instead become associated with the French neurologist Désiré-Magloire Bourneville, while working as an assistant to the revered Jean-Martin Charcot, who first described the disease in a 15-year-old girl. Hence, also known as Bourneville disease, this multi-system genetic disease can cause benign tumours to grow on the brain or other vital organs such as the kidneys, heart, eyes, lungs, and skin and results from mutations in other tumour suppressor genes, in a similar way to neurofibromatosis.

Another different tumour suppressor gene, when mutated, leads to increased cell production in various tissues and organs causing abnormal growth characteristic of the disease Proteus syndrome (*Proteus*; Greek God of the sea with an ability to change shape). Children with this disorder are usually born with normal appearance but develop tumours in the form of skin and bone growths as they age. Joseph Merrick, known as the *Elephant Man*, is suspected to have suffered from this disorder. There are suggestions a sister of his also inherited the condition. Born in Leicester in 1862 growths started erupting on his skin around the age of two. His disfigurement worsened as he grew older and, after his mother died, he was thrown out of the house. He would earn money exhibiting himself before the revered surgeon, Frederick Treves, organised a place for him to live at the London Hospital. Some of the highest in society would come to meet him, including Queen Victoria, who were amazed to discover that he was intelligent, articulate and sensitive. He

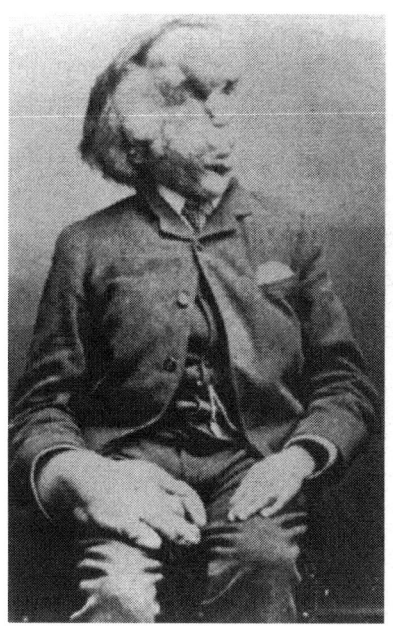

Joseph Merrick, 1889

showed that you cannot judge a person simply by their appearance. Dying in his sleep at
the age of 27 his skeleton is still displayed in the Royal London Hospital Museum.

*Tis true my form is something odd.*

*But blaming me is blaming God;*

*Could I create myself anew,*

*I would not fail in pleasing you.*

*If I could reach from pole to pole,*

*Or grasp the ocean with a span,*

*I would be measured by the soul,*

*The mind's the standard of the man.*

Isaac Watts (often quoted by John Merrick)

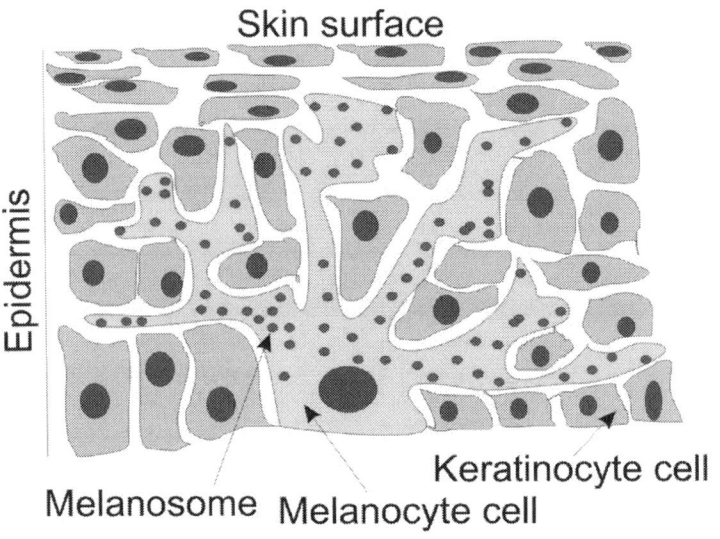

Skin surface

Epidermis

Keratinocyte cell

Melanosome  Melanocyte cell

Cross section of skin showing a melanocyte

Skin colour is chiefly the result of differing amounts of the pigment melanin (Gr. *melas*; black). This forms in little packets called melanosomes in special cells called melanocytes. These cells are found in the skin, eye and hair follicles and contain many branches which are used to move melanosome pigment packets they produce around to protect cells in the skin by absorbing harmful ultraviolet radiation preventing it reaching

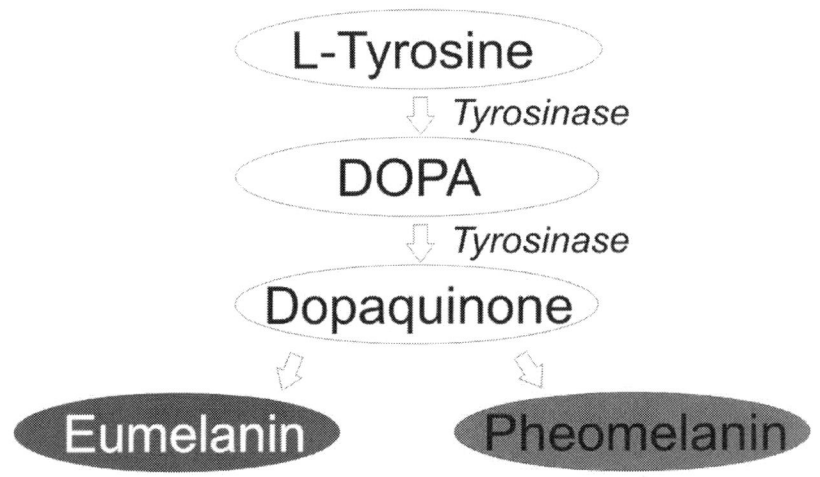

Melanin synthesis starts with phenylalanine being turned into tyrosine and further converted to dopa and then dopaquinone by the tyrosinase enzyme. This forms eumelanin or pheomelanin by two separate pathways

116

the DNA of the cells and causing mutations.

Pigment disorders can be caused by mutations in a variety of genes. Defects in the production of melanin pigment can be seen in oculocutaneous albinism. Defects in the formation of melanosomes occur in Hermansky-Pudlak syndrome. Defects in the development of melanocytes can lead to piebaldism, while a loss of melanocytes in later life leads to a condition known as vitiligo.

There are two types of melanin: the dark coloured eumelanin (Gr. *eu*; true) and the red-yellow pheomelanin (Gr. *Phaios*; brown/dusky). Both of these are formed from the amino acid tyrosine in a biochemical pathway involving a number of steps where one compound in a pathway is converted to the next compound by the action of an enzyme called tyrosinase.

Absence of either or both types of melanin leads to oculocutaneous (Lat. *oculus*; eye, *cutis*; skin) albinism (Lat. *albus*; white) (OCA). A complete lack of eumelanin and pheomelanin causes OCA1A where individuals are born with white skin and hair, and blue eyes, which remain throughout life. Photographs suggest that the musical brothers, Edgar

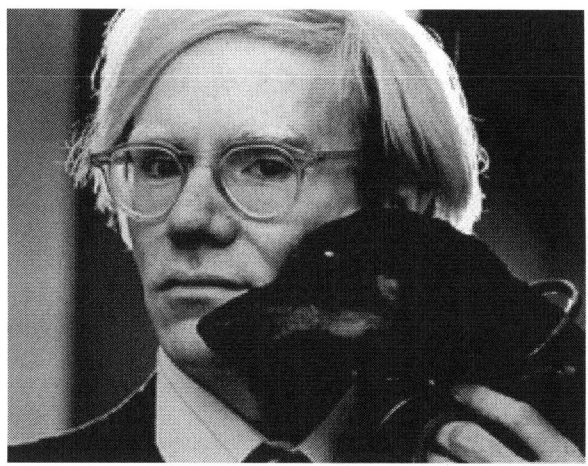

Andy Warhol, 1973

117

and Johnny Winter of the band *The Blues Brothers*, may have both inherited this form of albinism. Mutations that only reduce, but not completely remove, tyrosinase activity leads to OCA1B characterised by decreased levels of both types of melanin but the accumulation of a little pigment during ageing seen as the development of yellow hair with age. Some mutations lead to the enzyme working only in lower temperatures leading to the production of melanin only in cooler areas of the body, such as arms and legs, while warmer parts of the body, such as under the arms and the scalp, remain white. Photographs of Andy Warhol appear to show this.

Individuals with OCA3 lack the ability to produce melanin and are only able to generate red pheomelanin. These individuals have reddish skin, ginger/red hair, and brown eyes. This is quite common in the South African population where it is known as "Rufous". In the Bible a description of Esau suggests that he may have been born with this form of albinism, *"And the first came out red, all over like a hairy garment; and they called his name Esau"*, Genesis 25:25. The American blues musician William Lee Perryman performed under his stage name of *Piano Red*, due to this disorder.

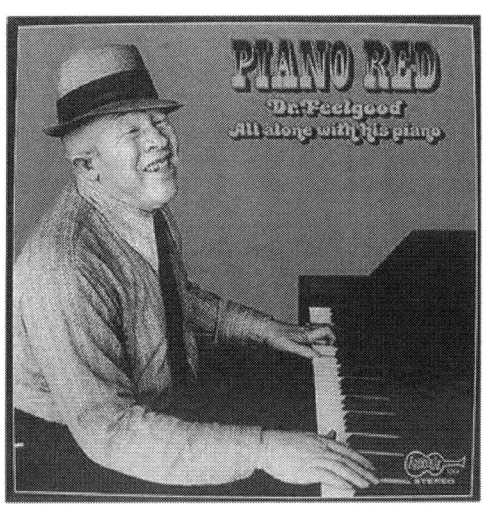

Album cover. *Piano Red: Dr. Feelgood All Alone With His Piano*, 1972

The most common type albinism is OCA2, resulting from mutations in a gene producing a protein involved in transporting molecules into and out of melanosomes. Caucasians with OCA2 show white to yellow hair, blue-grey eyes, and white skin that does not tan on sun exposure while darker-skinned individuals generally also show yellow hair and light brown skin colour. Jamaican-born reggae star Winston Foster, uses the stage-name *Yellowman*; his light skin and natural pale blond hair may have derived from this form of albinism.

Bleeding disorders generally never appear with albinism except in the related immune-related disorders Hermansky-Pudlak syndrome and Chediak-Higashi syndrome. Both of these are very rare disorders with Hermansky-Pudlak syndrome affecting around 1 in 1,000,000 individuals worldwide, and only 500 cases of Chediak-Higashi syndrome on record. In the movie *Cold Mountain* (2003), there is a villain with albinism who, in addition to the white makeup and bleached hair, suffers frequent nosebleeds – a detail not included in the book. Both these syndromes result from mutations in genes producing proteins responsible for the production of organelles used to store blood-clotting factors in platelets and white blood cells as well as in melanosomes. Nose-bleeding is generally rare in albinism except in those two syndromes suggesting that the actor while researching the disorder and finding links between albinism and bleeding might have been referring to either of these syndrome and not general albinism associated with OCA. The medical complications associated with these two syndromes often require hospital treatments and so not best suited to a cowboy in the Wild West. This is perhaps an example of the need to carefully research disorders before making generalisations.

Piebaldism (magpie, a black and white bird) is characterised by distinct patches of skin and hair lacking pigment. This results from defects during embryonic development, of the migration of cells from to the skin where they divide to produce melanocyte cells. One famous case is that of George Alexander Gratton. Born in 1808 on the Caribbean island of St Vincent, he was bought as a baby by John Richardson to work in his circus in England. Treating him as his son Richardson was distraught when the boy died later in childhood and had him buried at the All Saints Church in Marlow in the same vault in which he himself was later laid to rest.

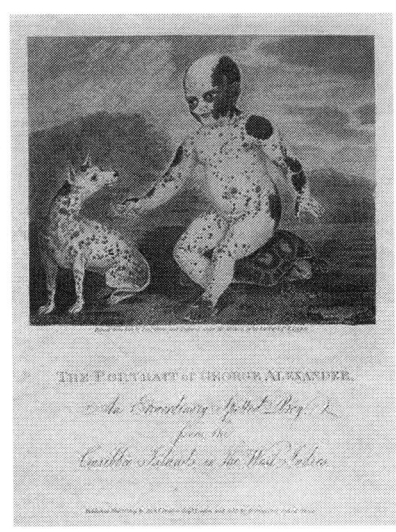

George Alexander Gratton by P.R. Cooper, 1809

Piebaldism can often present as very discrete depigmented patches of skin and hair. Autosomal dominantly inherited, generations with familial marks such as a white forelock have sometimes carried surnames as Whitlock, Horlick and Blaylock. There are a number of well-known people with distinct patches of pigment-less skin or hair. British politicians and brothers, David and Ed Miliband, for example, both have a small tuft of white hair in a similar area towards the front of their heads suggesting perhaps some shared gene.

In vitiligo (Gr. *vitelius*; calf, describing white patches on a cow) there is a destruction of melanocyte cells through an autoimmune reaction leading to patches of skin lacking pigment. This generally appears in adulthood but does not follow a simple inheritance pattern suggesting the involvement of a combination of multiple genes in addition to environmental factors. This condition is often unnoticeable on Caucasian skin. For instance, the Irish comedian Graham Norton's patches of depigmentation are not so apparent on the screen. However, on darker- skinned people, it is much more obvious. This condition affected Michael Jackson, his father and paternal grandfather suggesting a genetic inheritance. Such melanin-free patches of skin are sensitive to the sun, which is the reason Michael Jackson gave for often covering up his skin and wearing gloves outside. The Canadian supermodel Winnie Harlow, who has had this condition since the age of 4, serves as a spokesperson for this condition.

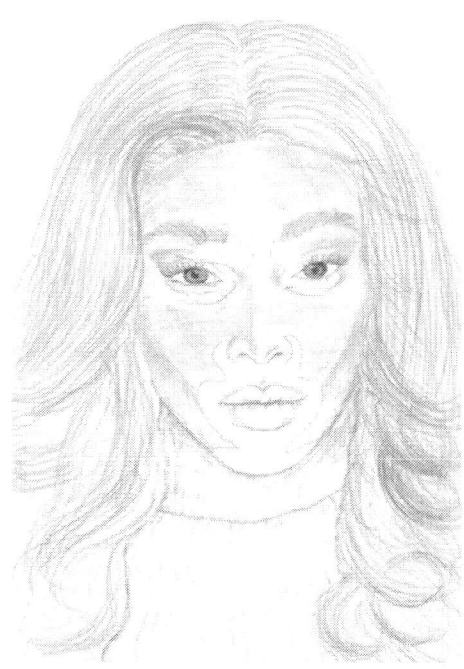

Winnie Harlow

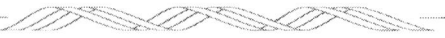

# HAIR DISORDERS

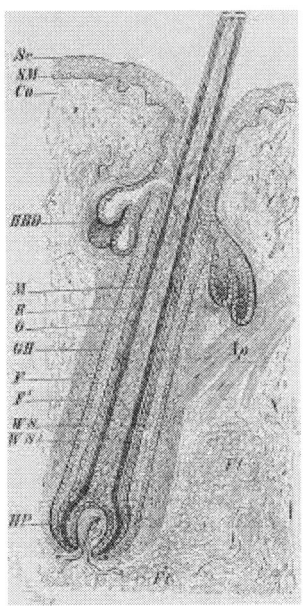

*What's so brave about being bald? I've not fought for my country or found the cure for cancer - I've just gone out without my hat on!*

Gail Porter

At the base of a hair, there are follicle cells expressing high amounts of keratin proteins. These cells multiply and push upward and die, to form the shaft of the hair. The three types of hair produced by the body are lanugo, vellus and terminal. Terminal hairs are found on the scalp, pubic area and other body areas such as the armpits. Vellus hair is the very fine light, almost invisible hair covering most of our bodies. Lanugo hair is found only in utero, covering the developing foetus and shed before birth. A number of genetic disorders associate with different patterns of hair loss, known as alopecia, hair overgrowth, called hypertrichosis, or alterations in hair structure causing fragile and twisted hair.

The most common cause of loss of head hair is androgenic alopecia, also known as male-pattern baldness. Androgenetic alopecia (Gr. *alopex*; fox – an animal that frequently suffers hair loss) results from alterations in male hormones (androgens), that cause hair follicles in the scalp to decrease in size later in life. The role of androgens, such as testosterone, in hair loss probably first became evident from the fact that eunuchs never seemed to go bald. Women also only rarely develop androgenic alopecia, though in the cases of abnormally high levels of testosterone, they not only go bald but also tend to grow beards, a condition known as hirsutism. In males, this condition is highly heritable and there are a few genes implicated. One of these is the androgen receptor gene on the X

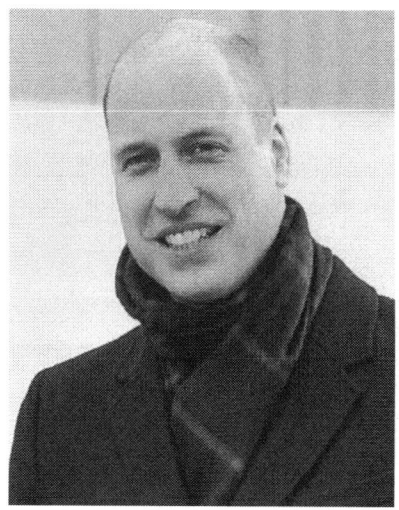

Prince William, 2018

chromosome, which may give some support to the wives' tales that male-pattern baldness comes from the mother's side of the family if this is X-linked inherited. However, it is certainly not the only gene involved, and there are a number of other genes and environmental factors.

Alopecia areata describes the loss of discrete regions of hair from the scalp and alopecia areata totalis is a term used if all scalp hair is lost in a relatively short time and at a relatively young age. The loss of all hair on the head and body, usually quite early in life, is known as alopecia universalis. Around 1 in 5 cases show inheritance in family members and they are generally thought to result from an autoimmune reaction whereby hair follicles, are damaged by a misguided immune system. Pierluigi Collina, the Italian football referee, suffered from this losing all his hair in the space of just two weeks when he was 24. The Swedish model Therese Hansson, first started losing her hair when she was just 14 years old, while Scottish television presenter, Gail Porter, developed the condition at the age of 34, losing much of her hair in a matter of just days. Refusing to wear a hat or wig, she has

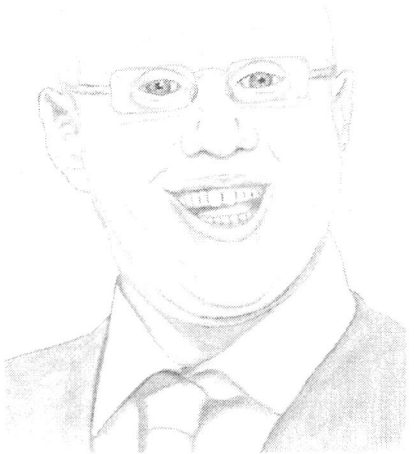

Matt Lucas

been able to raise important awareness of this condition in women. The British actor and comedian Matt Lucas, lost every hair on his body around the age of 6. His father also lost his hair at the age of 12 suggesting an inheritance.

The production of too much hair is known as hypertrichosis (Gr. *hyper*, excess, *trichos*; hair) and sometimes informally known as werewolf syndrome. One form of this disorder, known as hypertrichosis lanuginose, results in lanugo hair remaining on all parts of the body following birth. Lanugo hair is grown in utero and lost before birth, except in this genetic condition where the hair keeps on growing throughout life. One of the first recorded cases was of a boy called Petrus Gonzalez, covered from head to toe in soft lanugo hair. Born on Tenerife in 1556 he was "presented" to the French King, Henry II. He went on to marry and raise several children, some of whom also shared his condition, supporting an autosomal dominant inheritance pattern. However, a gene for this disorder has yet to be identified. Many people in the past with this condition have ended up being displayed like wild animals at circuses and sideshows. For example, Fedor Jeftichew, known as *Jo-Jo the*

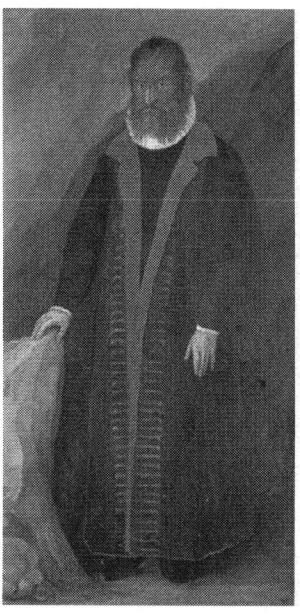

Petrus Gonzalez, anonymous, 1850

125

*Dog-Faced Boy* was born in St. Petersburg in 1868 to a father with the same condition. As part of a circus act, the story was that a hunter found him and his father in a cave as savages, and they could not be tamed, at which point he would growl at the audience who were oblivious to the fact that he was perfectly fluent in several languages. Born with this condition in China in 1849, Su Kong Tai Djin was abandoned as a baby in a forest to die by his family. However, a Shaolin monk travelling through the forest discovered him lying amongst the trees and took him back to a Shaolin Temple where he was raised by monks who taught him martial arts. Proving to be exceptionally gifted, he quickly became a favourite of many of the Shaolin masters from other temples in the area who each passed their knowledge on to him. Subsequently, he became the first Grandmaster of Shaolin and the first to master all skills of the seven Shaolin temples, including over 200 different empty hand systems, over 140 weapon systems, and specialities such as the infamous Death Touch. Still revered around the world, he lived until the age of 79 and taught many others to be masters.

Born in Mexico in 1854, Julia Pastrana was sold into marriage by her mother to Theodor Lent who exhibited her around the world in various circuses as *The Ape Woman*. This was due to a condition Julia was born with resulting in uncontrolled growth of dark terminal hair over her body. It would appear she had inherited a gene for hypertrichosis terminalis. Unknown to many, she was a highly intelligent woman who spoke several languages and was an accomplished musician with a beautiful voice. At the age of 26 years old she gave birth to a boy with the same disorder, but sadly he lived only thirty-five hours and Julia Pastrana herself died five days later. Her husband, however, had the bodies of his wife and son mummified and carried on exhibiting them. Incredibly, during one of the tours, Theodor met and married another woman with a similar condition to Julia whom he introduced during his acts as Zenora Pastrana a sister of Julia. Sometime later Theodor Lent suffered a mental breakdown and died in an asylum, while Zenora continued touring with the mummies before selling them to the owner of a shop of oddities in Oslo. The bodies then fell into Nazi hands, where they again went on tour around Europe, and then in the U.S. after the war. They were rediscovered in a basement in the Oslo Forensic Institute in 1990. However, scientists refused to give the bodies up and obtained a special permit to conduct research. Finally, in 2012, the Sinaloa state governor was able to secure the return of her body and hundreds of people attended her Catholic funeral, as her remains were finally buried in a cemetery in Sinaloa de Leyva, close to her birthplace.

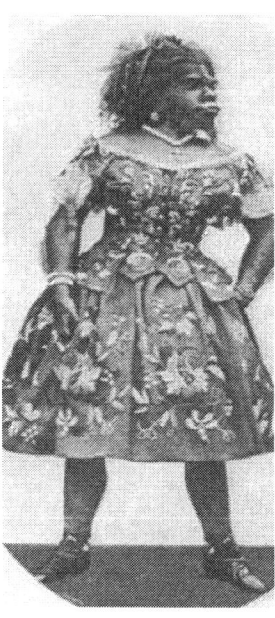

The embalmed body of Julia Pastrana, 1900

There are some genetic conditions in which the shape of hair can be disrupted. Uncombable hair syndrome is a condition that is characterised by dry, frizzy hair that cannot be combed flat. Caused by mutations in genes that provide instructions for making proteins that help give structure to the hair shaft, the condition usually develops early in

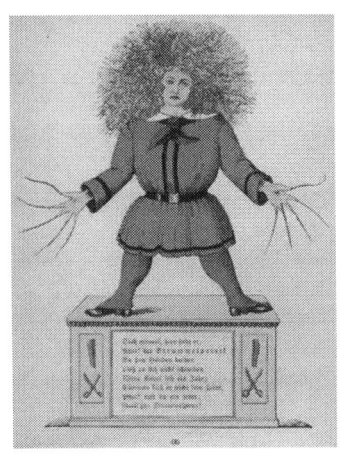

*Der Struwwelpeter*, by Heinrich Hoffmann, 1917

life. This disorder is also known as Struwwelpeter syndrome after the bushy-haired character *Shockheaded Peter* from the 19th-century German children's book *Der Struwwelpeter*. Some speculate that Einstein may have had this condition.

Characteristic hair defects can be markers for a number of genetic diseases resulting from reductions in key components important for the structure of keratin proteins. Low levels of arginine underlie Sabinas Brittle Hair syndrome first observed in a small Mexican town called Sabinas. Genetic disruptions in the control of copper can lead to Menkes kinky hair syndrome highlighting the importance of Copper in hair formation.

Hair colour, like skin colour, derives from melanin. A lack of melanin, as seen in albinism, results in white hair, while a loss of hair colour during older age is known as canities (Lat. *canus*; grey) and the appearance of white hairs in early adulthood is known as premature greyness. The appearance of white hair at specific locations, such as a white forelock, may sometimes associate with a number of genetic disorders, such as Piebaldism and Waardenburg syndrome. This is sometimes known as a Mallen stripe and is associated with witches; think of *Cruella de Vil, Bellatrix Lestrange, Lily Munster* and the *Bride of Frankenstein*. The term 'Mallen streak' was coined in the 1970s by the novelist Catherine Cookson in her

'*Mallen*' books about a family who all shared the hereditary streak and came to no good. However, this stripe of white hair has had villainous connotation since medieval times. In order to lynch women as witches, numerous naturally occurring physical traits such as moles, birthmarks and a stripe of white hair, that came to be known as a 'Witch's Streak', were considered signs of evil. It is curious that some of these anomalies still seem to have kept their association with evil. This is especially evident in Halloween consumes, horror films and also some children's movies.

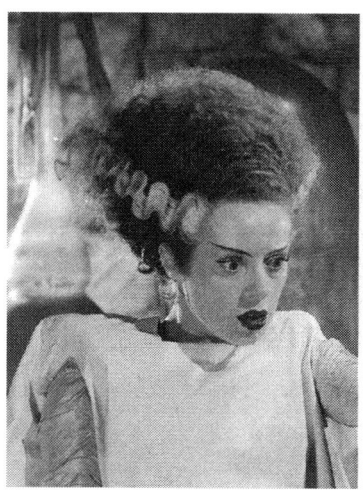

Elsa Lanchester in *Bride of Frankenstein*, 1935

Various shades of red hair result from differences in genes controlling melanin and pheomelanin. Alpha-Melanocyte-stimulating hormone (alpha-MSH) is a hormone that binds to receptors, such as the melanocyte-stimulating hormone receptor 1 (MC1R) on melanocytes, causing the cell to produce the dark pigment eumelanin. A lack of alpha-MSH results in the melanocytes not being stimulated and, instead, producing phaeomelanin leading to red or blond hair. The gene for the MC1R receptor has many different polymorphic forms differing in their activities which, in a variety of combinations, cause the different colours of hair from red, to auburn, to strawberry blond. A majority of the red-headed Celts have gene variants that produce receptors that are almost totally inactive. It is interesting that red hair is most commonly found in people of Scandinavian descent and it is thought that the clusters of redheads in the British Isles derive from Viking ancestry. Scotland has the highest proportion of redheads of any country with 13 per cent of the population having red hair and a further 40 per cent carrying the highly inactive MC1R variant gene. It may be that the high occurrence or red-hair, particularly in northern Europe, is due to evolution selecting for red-headed people. One theory is that this might be due to their accompanying lighter skin allowing them to absorb more sunlight for vitamin D production.

As well as binding to the MC1R receptor, alpha-MSH also binds to another similar receptor called MC4R; this is important for regulating appetite. A small number of people have a genetic deficiency of alpha-MSH causing red hair and reduced control of appetite, leading to obesity in some in individuals. However, this only affects a small proportion of redheads as most red-haired individuals have alterations in the alterations in the MC1R gene receptor and not a lack of alpha-MSH.

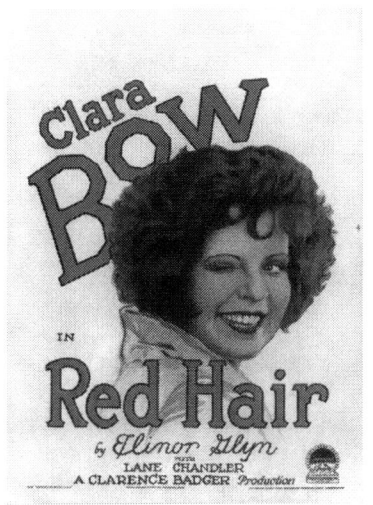

Poster for the film *Red Hair*, 1928

# RESPIRATORY DISORDERS

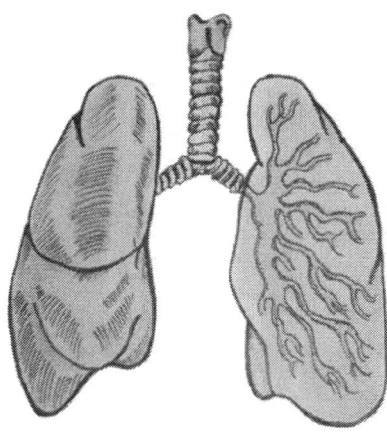

*Sometimes I can only groan, suffer, and pour out my despair at the piano!*

Chopin

Lungs deliver oxygen to the body, remove carbon dioxide waste, regulate temperature and stabilise blood pH balance. To prevent lung tissues from drying out and to prevent infections, mucus is produced consisting of proteins, salts and immune system components suspended in water. Increased mucus production in the respiratory tract is stimulated in response to many diseases, such as the common cold. However, one disease called cystic fibrosis results in the mucus becoming too viscous, therefore impeding breathing.

Superstition in the Middle Ages held that infants with salty skin would die an early death. It was a common practice to lick the forehead of a child to taste for the presence of salt and the occurrence of this disease. This would have related to cystic fibrosis, the most common autosomal recessive disorder in Europeans affecting around 1 in 2,500 births in the UK. This disease results from a mutation in a gene producing a protein that allows cells to move chloride ions (which, along with sodium, makes up salt) into and out of the cells. This is important to maintain an osmotic balance between the inside and outside of cells. This mutation disrupts the ability of this protein to function leading to increased chloride ions in the cells lining the windpipe and intestines which draws water from the mucus dehydrating and thickening it. This thick mucus then clogs the lungs causing breathing problems and infections and also impairs the ability of the intestines that depend upon mucus to aid digestion.

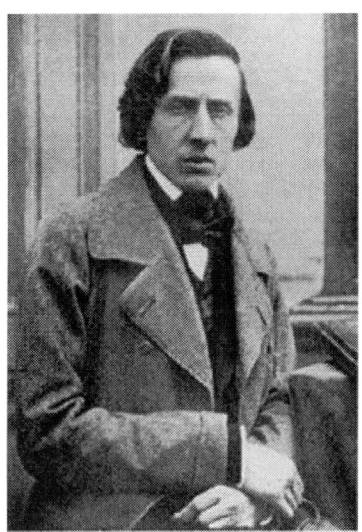

Frédéric Chopin, 1847

It is thought Frédéric Chopin may have suffered from this. His frail health started early in childhood with recurrent diarrhoea and gastro-intestinal ailments resulting in weight loss, and frequent respiratory tract infections. He would often be confined to his bed for long periods, from where he would give his piano lessons in a lying position. Chopin's father and two of his sisters also suffered from respiratory problems possibly indicating a hereditary link. Another musician, British singer-songwriter, Alice Martineau suffered and died from cystic fibrosis at the age of 30. Thinking that her condition would prevent her from singing, Alice did not at first pursue her musical ambitions but she later discovered that her constant coughing had actually strengthened her vocal cords. She died shortly after releasing her debut album Daydreams in 2002.

To protect the lungs from infection there are white blood cells which release a powerful enzyme called elastase. This breaks down invading pathogens without damaging the delicate lung tissues which are protected by a second protein called alpha-1-antitrypsin that inactivates the elastase in the immediate vicinity of the lung tissue. Inheriting gene differences that disrupt this second protein can lead to lung damage and emphysema, known as alpha-1-antitrypsin deficiency. Inherited autosomal recessively and affecting around 1 in every 2,500 people, sufferers develop symptoms between the ages of 20 and 40 years old with a of shortness of breath and the development of emphysema (Gr. *emhysan*; inflate) caused by the destruction of their lung tissue. Some toxins, such as cigarette smoke, directly inactivate alpha-1-antitrypsin so speeding up the process of elastase-induced lung damage. People with different mutations in this gene can have differing degrees of susceptibility to toxins such as tobacco. This genetic link might have been responsible for the pattern of smoking-related illnesses in the family of Richard Reynolds, one of the founders of the cigarette industry. After years of smoking, he died of emphysema, followed by two of his four children, and many subsequent family members who also smoked. One of his grandchildren, Patrick Reynolds, is now a highly prominent anti-smoking activist in the US. In 2008 Amy Winehouse was diagnosed at the age of 24 with emphysema. Even though she smoked heavily, her very young age has led to some speculation that she may have some level of alpha-1-antitrypsin deficiency, though this has not been confirmed.

This phenomenon of inherited susceptibilities to certain toxins has been an issue in a number of court cases. One case in the 1970s involved the Dow Chemical Company that started testing prospective employees for alpha-1-antitrypsin deficiency claiming that they were trying to protect prospective alpha-1-antitrypsin deficient employees from industrial pollutants. The union argued that the testing was an unfair labour practice and maintained that the onus should be on the industry to make the workplace safe for everyone, regardless of their alpha-1-antitrypsin status. The company subsequently discontinued the tests.

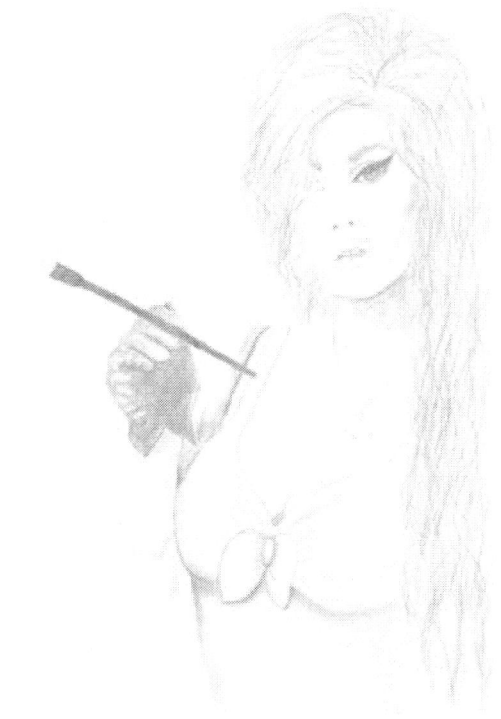

Amy Winehouse

# HEART DISORDERS

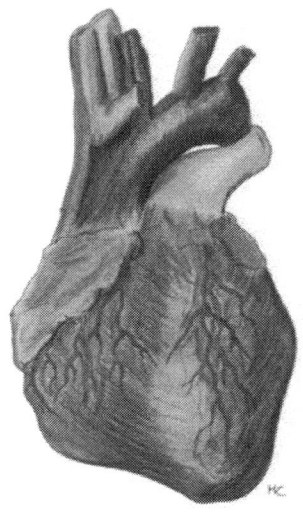

*Once I had brains, and a heart also; so having tried them both, I should much rather have a heart.*

The Tin Woodsman of Oz

Congenital heart defects, describe those present at birth. They affect almost 1 per cent of all babies born, and are the leading cause of birth defect-related deaths. These include a variety of malformations of the heart or its major blood vessels that may obstruct blood flow or cause blood to flow through the heart in an abnormal pattern.

While the cause of most congenital heart defects is unknown, some heart malformations do have a clear genetic link such as from large chromosome aberrations occurring in 22q11.2 deletion syndrome, and single gene defects as seen in syndromes such as Noonan syndrome. In addition, a vast and diverse number of genetic syndromes also present with heart defects as one of the symptoms.

Affecting 1 in 1,000-2,500 births the autosomal dominant inherited Noonan syndrome is one of the most common conditions associated with congenital heart anomalies. Resulting from mutations in a gene encoding a protein important in regulating cell growth and formation of the heart valves, individuals have heart defects, short stature, learning problems, an indentation of the chest, impaired blood clotting, and characteristic facial features. It has been suggested that the blacksmith in the famous painting, *Among Those Left* by the American artist Ivan Le Lorraine Albright, had Noonan syndrome judging from the contour of the breastbone, the low-set ears, and short stature.

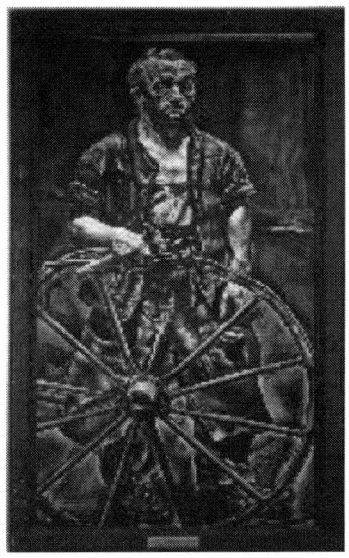

*Among those left* by Ivan Albright, 1928

Tetralogy of Fallot is a heart anomaly named after the French physician Étienne-Louis-Arthur Fallot, that refers to a combination of four (Gr. *tetra*, four) related heart defects present at birth that affect the structure of the heart and cause oxygen-poor blood to flow out of the heart and to the rest of the body. Infants and children with tetralogy of Fallot usually have blue-tinged skin as their blood does not carry enough oxygen. This is sometimes known as blue baby syndrome. Affecting 1 in 2,000 births, it is often associated with 22q11.2 deletion syndrome, though can also occur through a number of different single-gene mutations, as well as some environmental factors.

The Dutch painter Dick Ket was believed to have suffered from this. His numerous self-portraits show another characteristic, often seen in this disease, which is a progressive enlargement of the fingers, known as clubbing, due to reduced levels of oxygen reaching these parts of the body. Even after successful surgery, patients with tetralogy of Fallot face a greater risk of serious heart problems. They need regular check-ups to monitor their heart throughout their lifetime. However, this does not necessarily mean individuals are unable to

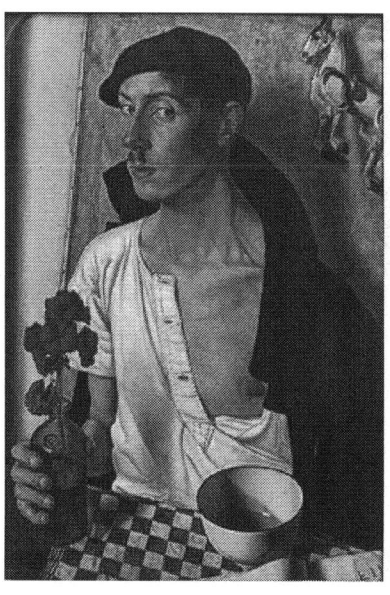

Dick Ket, *self-portrait*, 1932

lead an active life. The snowboarding legend Shaun White was also born tetralogy of fallot, for which he underwent two open-heart operations when he was one year old. Professional skateboarder and snowboarder he holds the record for the most X-Games gold medals and most Olympic gold medals by a snowboarder. The Australian test cricketer, Beau Casson likewise underwent open heart surgeries at a young age for the same condition.

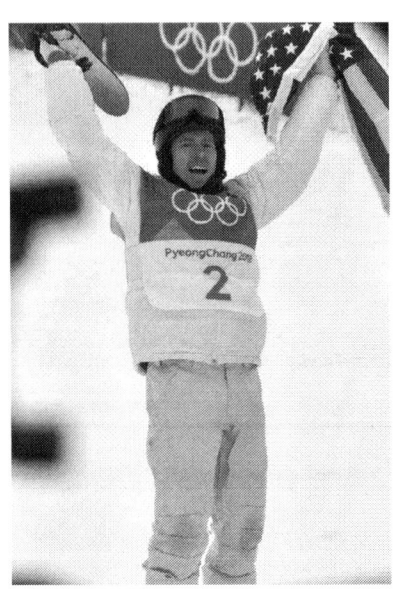

Shaun White, Winter Olympics, 2018

The loss of a large part of chromosome 22 containing around 30 genes leads to heart defects and an opening in the roof of the mouth known as a cleft palate. Occurring in around 1 in 1,800 births, the features of this syndrome are so varied that it has been given a number of different names such as DiGeorge syndrome and Shprintzen syndrome by researchers who were convinced that they had discovered a new syndrome. However, once it became clear that these symptoms were all determined by the same chromosome 22 deletion, they were grouped into a single syndrome. It then became known for a while as CATCH22 (for cardiac abnormality, T-cell deficit, clefting and hypocalcaemia, chromosome 22). Although a clever title, it obviously has serious negative overtones with some parents perhaps finding themselves in such a situation, and so fell out of favour. It is now known more prosaically as 22q11.2 deletion syndrome.

In addition to the major congenital heart defects diagnosed at birth, as many as a further 1 in 150 babies in the UK are born with heart defects that often go undiagnosed initially because they are not associated with any other accompanying symptoms. Sudden infant death syndrome (SIDS), also known as cot death, occurs in around 200 babies in the UK each year. Although the causes of most cases of SIDS are not clear, underlying heart defects appear to have a role in a significant percentage of cases. Over 200 women in the UK have been convicted of the murder or mistreatment of one or more of their infants who died without a known cause, i.e. SIDS. The British paediatrician, Sir Roy Meadows, who was involved in the prosecution of many of these women, famously asserted *"one cot death is a tragedy, two is suspicious and three is murder"*. He calculated there to be a 1 in 73 million probability that a mother could have three children dying of cot deaths and this was a major factor in persuading juries to arrive at a guilty verdict in the trials of these women. This calculation completely ignores any possible genetic links, which obviously greatly increase the risk of SIDS in a particular family. It also ignores environmental factors such as bacterial infections, mould spores, and having a parent who smokes, which also greatly increase risks. Many of these unsafe convictions have since been overturned.

One particular abnormality, that studies suggest affects up to a third of SIDS, is a prolongation of the QT interval in the first week of life. The QT interval is the length of time it takes the electrical system to recharge following a heartbeat. A percentage of infants dying of SIDS in the first week of life show a prolongation of the QT interval. In some cases, there are underlying genetic mechanisms and a large number of different inherited long QT syndromes have been identified resulting from different mutant genes. For example, one mutant gene for a potassium channel is suspected to underlie around a third of all genetic cases. Potassium ions are necessary for the electrical conduction system of the heart. This defect can also leave an individual with a vulnerability to suddenly developing a very fast, abnormal heart rhythm in adulthood, known as sudden arrhythmic syndrome. In such an instance no blood is pumped out of the heart causing sudden death, This affected the Manchester City midfielder Marc-Vivien Fóe who collapsed and died on June 26th 2003 in the 72nd minute of the Confederations Cup semi-final between Cameroon and Columbia. No other player was within five yards of him.

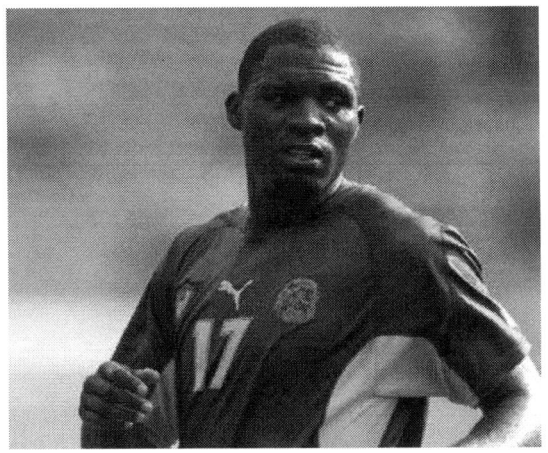

Marc-Vivien Foé, 2003

It is not clear how many young athletes suddenly die in adulthood from heart abnormalities, though an Italian study suggested a figure of around in 1 in 50,000 a year. Over a period of 10 days in the summer of 2007 several footballers suffered heart attacks, sending shock waves around the sporting world. On August 16th Leicester City player, Clive Clarke, suffered a heart attack during a League Cup tie at Nottingham Forest, though he recovered in hospital. Four days later Walsall's 16-year-old youth-team player Anton

Reid suddenly collapsed and died on the training ground. Then on the 28th August the Seville left-back, Antonio Puerta, suffered a fatal heart attack followed less than 24 hours later by Chaswe Nsofwa, a Zambia international, who died during training. Later in the year the Motherwell captain Phil O'Donnell collapsed and died during his team's game against Dundee United.

While long QT syndrome has been identified in a number of cases, the leading cause of sudden death in people under the age of 30, is an inherited heart condition known as hypertrophic cardiomyopathy. This results in the build-up of an abnormal protein inside heart muscle cells causing the muscles to thicken and the heart to develop an irregular beat. Currently, 9 genes are known to cause the disorder, coding for proteins in heart muscle cells. Around 1 in 500 people are born with hypertrophic cardiomyopathy through many show no symptoms, often going undetected. They nevertheless have a 1% chance of sudden death each year. Daniel, the son of former Wales's football manager Terry Yorath, suddenly died from this condition during a kick-about with his father in their garden. He was 15 years old and had just signed for Leeds United. Miklos Feher, Benfica's 24-year-old striker, was already well into his footballing career before this disease claimed his life during a 2004 league clash against Vitoria Guimaraes.

As excessive exercise can be a trigger for sudden death in otherwise healthy people with undetected heart defects a number of sport regulatory bodies have compulsory medical checks for athletes. The football federation, FIFA, driven by the tragic death of Marc Vivien Foé and others, implemented a number of initiatives to help prevent and raise awareness about sudden cardiac arrest in football players. In 2006, FIFA standardised the pre-competition medical assessment to include the detection of cardiovascular anomalies and provision of response training for referees, sports scientists, players and staff.

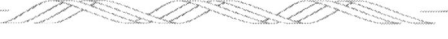

# LIVER DISORDERS

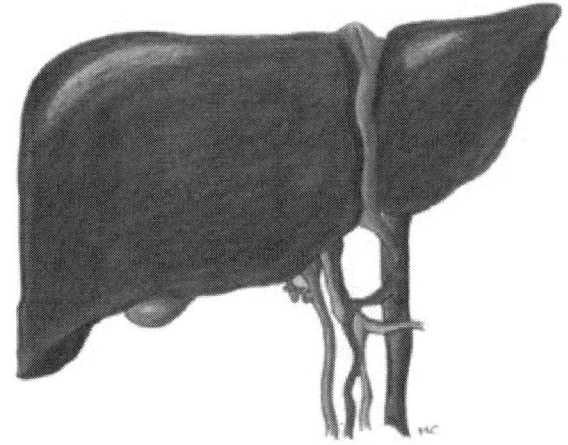

*Don't die like me.*

George Best

The liver receives blood directly from the intestines containing almost everything absorbed by the gut, including nutrients, drugs, and sometimes toxins. This flows through a latticework of tiny channels inside the liver, where the digested nutrients and toxins are processed. The liver is the only organ in the body which can regrow if part of it is removed. This allows surgeons to be able to cut out cancerous part of the liver leaving a small amount behind to regenerate. In Greek mythology, *Prometheus* was punished by the gods for

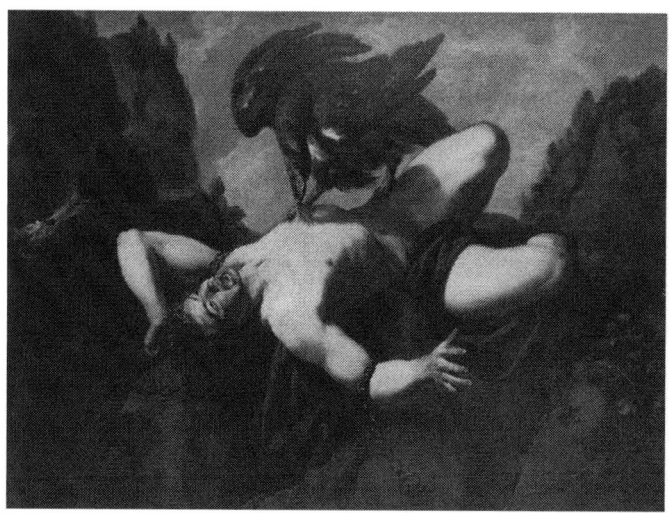

*Prometheous*, Theodoor Rombouts, 1597–1637

revealing fire to humans by being chained to a rock where a vulture would peck out his liver, which would grow again overnight only to be eaten again when the eagle returned the following morning. How the ancient Greeks knew about the liver's regenerative capacity is a mystery.

Symptoms of liver disease can include abdominal pains, vomiting and jaundice where the skin turns a yellowish colour due to the accumulation of bile pigments in the blood that is normally removed by the liver. When chronic diseases cause the liver to become permanently injured and scarred, the condition is called cirrhosis. The Football legend George Best died from this in 2005 due to his alcoholism. The British tabloid *News of the World* carried out his final request of publishing a picture of him in his hospital bed along with a message: *"Don't die like me"*.

Wilson's disease results from mutations in a gene disrupting the ability of the liver to move copper to the bile for excretion. Instead, it builds up in the liver and is released into the blood depositing throughout the body, particularly in the kidneys, eyes and brain leading to psychiatric symptoms in addition to liver disease. With symptoms tending to develop in late teens and or early twenties, it affects around one in 35,000 people. Treatment involves reducing the amount of copper accumulating in the body by taking chemicals that bind the copper and drugs that reduce the gut's ability to absorb copper. However, liver transplantation is sometimes needed if the liver becomes too damaged. This happened to Howard Dell, a former Olympic bob-sleigher, professional basketball and football player, decathlete, trainer of Olympic athletes, and actor in *The Young and The Restless, That 70s Show, LA Heat* and *Totally Blonde*. After years of ignoring symptoms, he was given just months to live after he finally went to a hospital in 2006. But a quick liver transplant enabled him to recover and he is now regular gold medallist in the Canadian Transplant Games and World Championships. As the copper can also accumulate within the nervous system, neurological symptoms can also occur, including tremors, involuntary movements and difficulties in swallowing and speaking. A student in the UK, Alicia Goss, has been raising awareness of this. At University she began to lose her ability to walk straight and started to slur her speech. Many people assumed she was drunk until she was diagnosed and prescribed treatment. Her story was reported in some newspapers when she got the hospital to issue her a special card explaining her condition so she could get past nightclub bouncers who would previously deny her entry assuming she was drunk.

In 1928, the physician Dr Clarence Hemingway, after arriving home from work, shot himself. He is known to have developed bronze diabetes in his later life, a condition describing a pigmentation of the skin. This results from deposition of excess iron that

144

stimulates melanin production, together with diabetes. The iron can also affect the brain and he developed depression and memory loss in the years prior to his suicide at the age of 59. Thirty-three years later, his son Ernest Hemmingway would also kill himself at the age of 61 after showing very similar symptoms. Five members of the Hemingway family over four generations committed suicide, including his sister Ursula, his brother Leicester and his granddaughter Margaux. All of these probably had the same highly-treatable disease

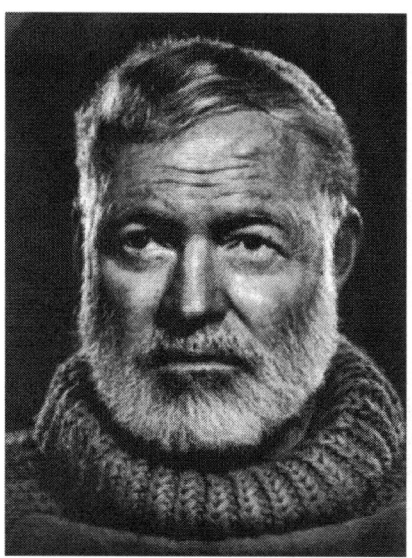

Ernest Hemingway, 1956

known as haemochromatosis. Indeed, medical records show that Ernest was diagnosed with this months before his death. In this disease individuals accumulate high levels of iron in their bodies that can lead to liver damage, diabetes mellitus and congestive heart failure; most only develop symptoms over the age of 50 years old. This is one of the most common genetic diseases, affecting as many as 1 in 200. This syndrome has also been reported in the family of another great American author, John Steinbeck, whose son John Steinbeck IV, also an author, was affected. Fascinatingly, there is still discussion over whether the excess levels of accumulated iron in this disorder can set off metal detectors in airports.

Familial hypercholesterolemia, affecting as many as 1 in 500 people, is characterised by high levels of cholesterol in the blood. Produced in the body and obtained from foods that come from animals, such as eggs and meat, we need cholesterol to build cell membranes, make certain hormones, and produce compounds that aid in fat digestion. Too much cholesterol, however, increases a person's risk of developing heart disease as it deposits in the walls of blood vessels. A common defect underlying this is in the gene producing the low-density lipoprotein receptor. This binds to particles called low-density lipoproteins, which are the primary carriers of cholesterol in the blood thus removing these from the bloodstream. Individuals with this defect have an increased risk of heart attacks and heart disease. Cholesterol may also be deposited in yellowish patches around the eyelids and form lumps in the tendons of the hands, elbows, knees and feet.

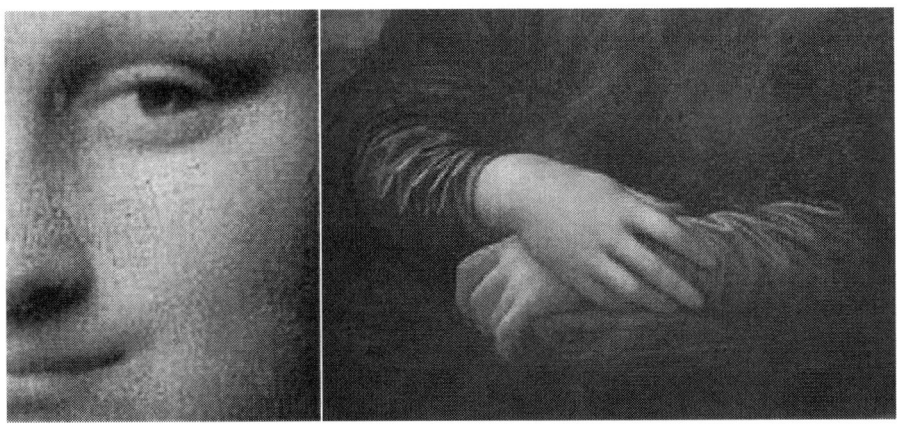

*Mona Lisa*, Leonardo da Vinci, 1503

Leonardo da Vinci, in addition to his art, is famed for his remarkable efforts in scientific work and anatomical investigations. Careful clinical examination of the *Mona Lisa* reveals a yellow irregular leather-like spot at the inner end of the left upper eyelid and a well-defined swelling on the right hand beneath the index finger. This may be the first depicted case of this disease.

The liver is involved in the breakdown of the haemoglobin component of red blood cells into bile pigments (bilirubin and biliverdin) that are excreted by the liver into the bile duct and through the bowels. High circulating levels of bile pigments in the blood can lead to the skin, and the whites of the eyes, showing a yellow colour known as jaundice. The urine can also appear darker as the pigments pass through the kidneys. Inherited defects in a gene coding for a liver enzyme involved in the processing and solubilising the bile pigment, bilirubin, causes Gilbert's syndrome. This can present with intermittent jaundice, particularly in times of illness, stress, exertion, poor diet or consumption of liver toxins such as excessive alcohol. However, this very common hereditary condition is usually harmless with some studies suggesting lower risks of coronary heart disease in affected individuals. British comedian, Noel Fielding has explained that if he drinks too much alcohol, he gets slight jaundice as a result of this disorder.

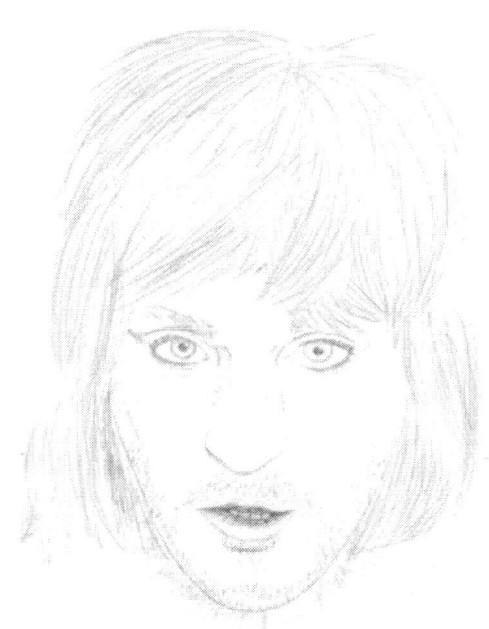

Noel Fielding

# KIDNEY DISORDERS

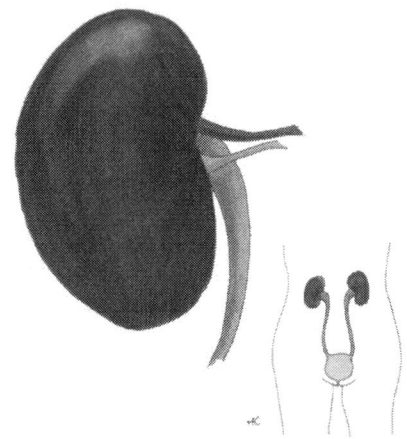

*It's what you do for your mates.*

Grant Kereama, Jonah Lomu's kidney donor.

The main job of the kidney is to filter waste products and excess fluid from the blood, excreting this as urine. They form two bean-shaped organs, except in around 0.2% of the population where the kidneys are fused into a single horseshoe-shaped structure; a condition which the actor Mel Gibson has. Early childhood kidney diseases often cause short stature due to the imbalance of salts and acids reducing appetite and preventing calcium being deposited in bones. Gary Coleman, the child star of *Different Stokes* fame, was born with a congenital kidney disease as a result of an autoimmune reaction. This restricted his growth leading to his shortened stature of 142 cm.

The ailments of *Tiny Tim* in Charles Dickens's novel *The Christmas Carol* is suggestive of a childhood kidney disorder known as Renal tubular acidosis. As well as short stature, this results crippling weakness, kidney stones and untimely death if left untreated. Caused by the kidneys failing to excrete acids into the urine, the treatment generally includes sodium bicarbonate to neutralise the acids in the blood. This treatment may well have been what *Ebenezer Scrooge* purchased for *Tiny Tim* in the story. Dickens had a keen interest in medical disorders and included many characters in his novels, with disorders and conditions that he had observed among friends and acquaintances. *Tiny Tim* was supposedly based on the invalid son of a friend who owned a cotton mill in Ardwick, Manchester.

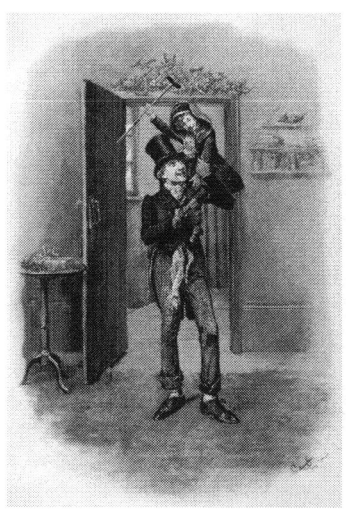

*Bob Cratchit and Tiny Tim,* 1870s

In order to perform the task of filtering waste products from the blood, the kidney uses special membranes which act as selective barriers. Defects in these membranes can lead to kidney failure characterised by the presence of high concentrations of blood in the urine; this is called thin basement membrane disease. First described in male members of a British family by Dr Cecil Alport in 1927, most cases result from defects in a gene on the X chromosome, explaining why males are more commonly affected. This symptom of blood in the urine occurred in the US president, Chester Alan Arthur, in 1882, along with fatigue and irritability. Shortly later, and just a year into his presidency, he was diagnosed with kidney disease - a medical fact that was kept secret by Arthur's staff.

When the King of Poland, Stefan Bathory, died in 1585 at the age of 53, the surgeon who performed the autopsy described the kidneys as *"large like those of a bull with an uneven and bumpy surface"*. This would appear to be the first description of polycystic kidney disease. A common life-threatening genetic disorder, this results in the development of large numbers of cysts in the kidney that impair the ability of the kidney to function properly. The American humourist and news column writer, Erma Louise Bombeck, died from this disease at 69 years old. She was diagnosed aged 20 and endured daily dialysis. and years of

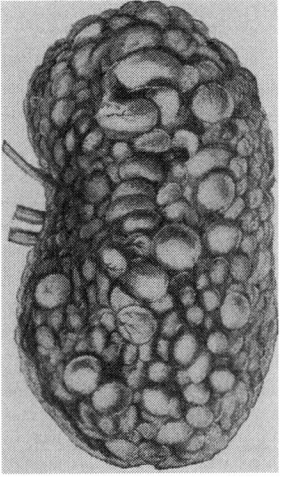

A drawing of polycystic kidney, 1893

150

wait for a transplant; one kidney had to be removed, and the remaining one ceased to function. In 1996, she received a kidney transplant but died a few weeks later from complications of the operation

In nephrosclerosis high blood pressure leads to a thickening of arteries in the kidney, reducing its ability to function properly. It is typically associated with high levels of proteins, particularly albumin, in the blood. The Russian writer Mikhail Bulgakov died of this kidney disease in 1940, suffering from the same symptoms as his father and dying at the same age of 48 years old, suggesting inheritance of a dominant gene. Educated as a medical doctor, it seems likely that Bulgakov realised he did not have long to live and so focussed himself on finishing his final novel, the political and satirical masterpiece, *The Master and Margarita*, which was critical of the Stalin regime and was immediately banned in his native Russia. A recent analysis of the original manuscript using mass-spectrometry detected several proteins known to be characteristic of the disease together with high levels of morphine that he took as a pain killer. The New Zealand All Black rugby legend Jonah Lomu was diagnosed with nephrotic syndrome, also characterised by high levels of proteins in the blood, aged 20 in 1995 not long after his first international cap. Amazingly he was able to still compete at

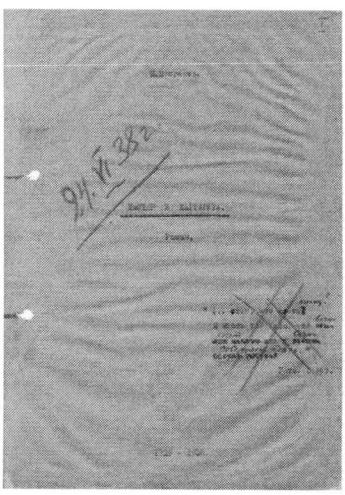

Cover page of the first typescript of Mikhail Bulgakov's novel the *Master and Margarita*

the highest level, but by 2003 he was on dialysis and in 2004 underwent a kidney transplant. Though making a comeback to professional rugby, he did not play international rugby again and died in 2015 after suffering a heart attack associated with his kidney condition while waiting for a second transplant. Jonah's cousin and All Black team-mate, Joeli Vidiri, also suffers from a kidney disease and currently undergoes regular dialysis.

In 2007, a Dutch TV company staged a competition *The Big Donorshow* where three contestants competed for the kidney of a dying woman. It quickly received widespread condemnation as being sick and unethical. Moments before the winner was revealed, as the floods of complaints poured in, they exclaimed it was 'partly' a hoax – the prospective donor was an actress. However, the three contestants were not actors; though in on the stunt they were nevertheless real kidney patients all desperately waiting for a transplant. In a direct response, was a sudden sharp rise in the number of people signing up to join the organ donor registry. It was no coincidence that the TV company screened this show on the fifth anniversary of the death of its founder and television star, Bart de Graaff, who died aged 35 after waiting many years for a kidney donation.

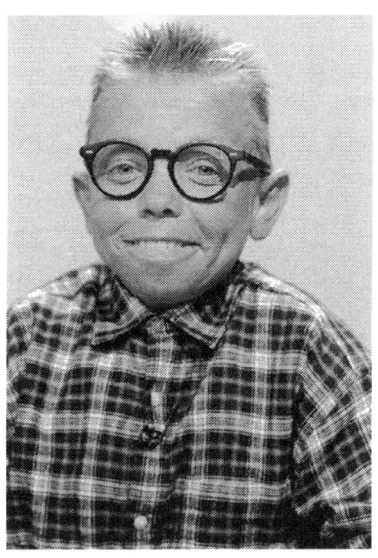

Bart de Graaff, 1991

# DIGESTIVE DISORDERS

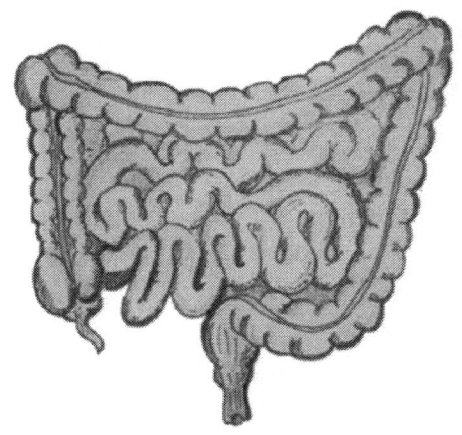

*There's nothing sexy about women saying: 'I've got to go to the bathroom right now'*

Shannen Doherty

The digestive system is made up of the digestive tract and other organs that help in digestive processes. Muscles in the stomach together with enzymes produced by stomach cells break down food particles, which then pass through the small intestine. Here other enzymes and other substances produced by cells in the small intestine, liver, and pancreas help in breaking down most of the food particles into smaller, easily absorbable substances. From here, nutrients and molecules are absorbed and transported by the blood to other parts of the body. The final process of digestion occurs in the large intestine, also known as the colon, through the activity of bacteria that live there.

The digestive system can be affected by many different conditions and diseases. Anatomical problems can arise as a result of a change in the shape of the digestive tract or the way it connects to other organs. Further diseases can result from a lack of particular enzymes, abnormalities in the bacterial flora, as seen in Crohn's disease, or reactions to certain substances that occur in Coeliac disease. Digestive problems may also occur when nerves controlling the digestive system are damaged, a condition called Hirschsprung's disease.

Crohn's disease is characterised by chronic inflammation of the intestines resulting in abdominal pain, diarrhoea, vomiting and weight loss. Affecting 1 in 5,000 people, it is caused by an overreaction to the digestive system's bacterial flora due to a lack of specific antibodies, known as defensins, which are secreted by the intestines. Though not strictly inherited, as it is multifactorial, it does tend to run in families and there are some genes that increase a person's risk, such as one that codes for one of the defensins. Dr Burrill Crohn, after whom the disease is named, recognised Crohn's as a particularly Jewish disease, reputedly joking that the ailment was brought on either by Jewish genes, Jewish food or Jewish mothers. Dwight D Eisenhower, the 34th President of the United States was diagnosed with Crohn's disease in 1956, six months before the presidential election. Again, presidential staff chose not to disclose information to the public until a severe inflammation of his intestine forced him to undergo surgery. Recovering from this, he won a second term as president. King Alfred the Great appeared to have possibly suffered and passed on a digestive disease, possibly Crohn's, to his grandson King Edred whose digestive malady proved so troublesome that towards the end of his life he would suck out the juices out of his food, chewed on what was left and spit it out.

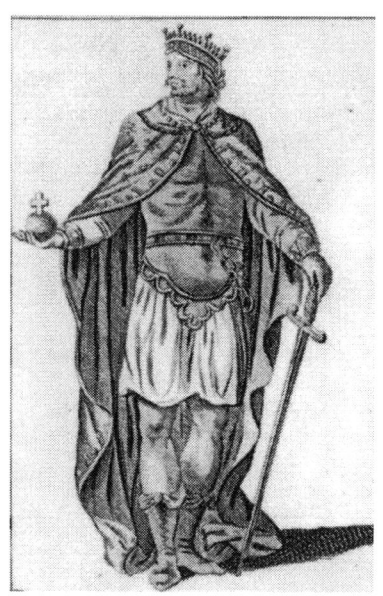

King Edred of England

Affecting around 1% of us, Coeliac disease (Gr; *koiliakós*, abdominal), results from an overreaction to gluten found in wheat, rye, malt, barley and oats in genetically predisposed individuals. This link was first noticed by Dr Willem Karel Dicke during the Dutch Famine of 1944 where with wheat in very short supply there was an improvement at a children's ward of coeliac patients. Exposure to these products damages the lining of the small intestine, reducing the ability to absorb nutrients. Though not strictly inherited, there is some genetic component with many sufferers inheriting one of two types of human leukocyte antigens involved in the immune system and autoimmunity. In many childhood cases the subsequent nutritional deficiencies can cause a range of symptoms such as diarrhoea, weight loss stunted growth and fatigue. Joe C, the sidekick of rock star Kid Rock, suffered from coeliac disease. This led to his reduced height and required him to undergo daily kidney dialysis until dying at the age of 26.

Louis Healy is an English actor who appears in the soup *Emmerdale* as *Danny Harrington*. The son of actors Tim Healy and Denise Walsh, he was born with a disease known as Hirschsprung's disease where nerve endings in the bowel do not form properly hindering the passage of digested food and stool. This can require an operation involving removing the affected part of the intestine lacking the normal nerve cells, and Louis indeed had a part of his large intestine removed at the age of 6 weeks and has made a full recovery. There are some genes involved with this disorder and there is an increased chance that a couple with one affected child will produce another baby with the disease. A number of mutated genes have been found that play roles in the development of neural cells in the digestive tract during embryonic development. However, Tim Healy and Denise Walsh's other son, Matthew, who is the lead singer of the British rock band *The 1975*, did not suffer any complications.

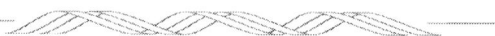

# BLOOD DISORDERS

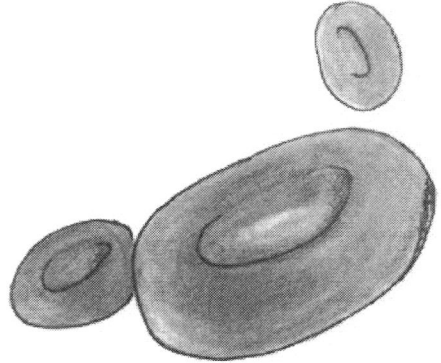

*How did we go from saving a child to evolution is dead?*

Parents of Molly Nash responding to Newspaper headlines.

Our red blood cells have a flattened shape with a depressed centre - biconcave. This optimises the exchange of oxygen and allows flexibility for the cells to fit through tiny capillaries. The average red blood cell travels around 1,000 miles through the maze of our body's circulatory system during its 120 days lifespan before being broken down in the spleen. Defects in the shape of these cells, such as in sickle cell anaemia and hereditary spherocytosis can lead to anaemia (Gr. *a*; absence, *haem*; blood).

In 1910, in Chicago, Walter Clement Noel, a 20-year-old dental student from Grenada, Caribbean, visited Dr James Herrick with complaints of pain episodes, and symptoms of anaemia. James passed on a sample of Walter's blood to a colleague, Dr Ernest Irons who, under the microscope, saw red blood cells he described as *"having the shape of a sickle"*. He published these findings giving the disease the name, sickle cell anaemia.

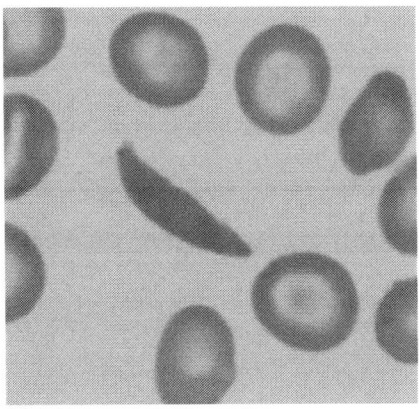

Normal and sickle-shape red blood cells

Although Noel was readmitted to hospital several times during his degree, he completed his studies returning to Grenada to practice dentistry. However, he died from the disorder shortly later, aged 27. This disorder appears to have been reported as far back as 5000 years ago in some parts of Africa with numerous names in different languages; in Nigeria the Igbo word *ogbanjes* meaning *"children who come and go"* due to the high infant mortality.

Caused by a specific mutation in a gene encoding one of the β-globin chains making up the haemoglobin protein complex, sickle-cell anaemia is one of the most common genetic disorders among Africans; around 1 in every 12 people is a carrier of the causal gene. In addition to African countries the disease has a high occurrence in many other countries where there are high incidences of malaria. This is due to a phenomenon known as heterozygous advantage, as individuals with only one mutant gene, carriers, though not suffering from sickle cell anaemia, show some resistance to malaria. This is because sickle cell carriers produce too small a number of sickle red blood cells to cause anaemia, but enough to give resistance to malaria. The malaria parasite, transmitted by mosquitoes, spends part of its life cycle in red blood cells which, in heterozygous sickle-cell anaemia carriers, results in the red blood cell rupturing leaving the parasite unable to reproduce. Therefore, heterozygotes in this area of the world have a greater evolutionary advantage.

Individuals with sickle cell anaemia tend to have problems from early life, although the severity can vary with some children showing few symptoms and being able to lead normal lives most of the time. The main problems of the sickle-shaped blood cells are that they can become stuck in small capillaries leading to severe pain. Sickle-shaped cells are also broken down more in the spleen and carry less oxygen leading to anaemia that can cause tiredness and shortness of breath.

There are a number of well-known musicians who have battled with this disease. Tionne Tenese "*T-Boz*" Watkins, the lead singer of the group *TLC* has described being in and out of hospital intensive care units since she was 7 years old with stays as long as four months. "*Sickle cell is very excruciating pain,*" she says. "*It feels like somebody is stabbing you over and over again*". Named one of *People* magazine's 50 Most Beautiful People in 2000, she is one of the spokespeople for the *Sickle Cell Disease Association of America*. Paul Williams, of the famed Motown group *The Temptations*, also suffered from this disease which drove him to alcohol. This however only worsens the symptoms as alcohol dehydrates leading to a thicker and reduced volume of blood that causes the sickle cells to clog even more, increasing the painful episodes. Eventually, on doctors' advice, he had to give up performing and in 1974, at the age of 34, was found dead next to his car with an, apparently self-inflicted, gunshot wound to the head. Miles Davis in 1961, aged 35, was diagnosed by a doctor as having sickle cell anaemia after suffering years of chronic joint pain. This may have been the

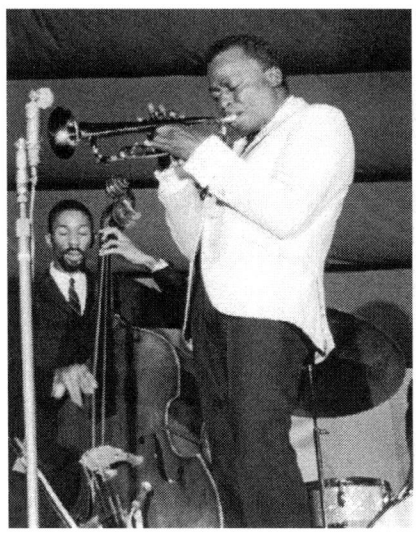

Miles Davis, 1963

reason he stopped playing jazz around this time, later referred to as his "silent period". Another symptom of the disease is that as blood flow is blocked in vessels supplying bone tissue, this tissue may die leading to increased fractures. The hip joint is particularly vulnerable. Miles Davis suffered numerous chipping of his bones in his wrists and had hip replacement operations though, incredibly, carried on performing until dying aged 65.

In the UK and the U.S. all babies are screened for sickle cell anaemia, in addition to phenylketonuria and a number of other disorders of metabolism, within the first 2 weeks of birth as part of the standard "heel-prick test" used to collect drops of blood. Although there is no cure, infants can be given painkillers, drugs to combat possible infections and advised to keep hydrated and warm.

Mutations in a number of different genes coding for membrane proteins can lead to red blood cells adopting a small spherical shape, known as Spherocytosis (*sphero*; spherical). These cells have less surface area to which oxygen can attach, but the main problem is that these misshapen but healthy red blood cells are mistaken by the spleen for old or damaged cells and are thus constantly being broken down by the spleen. This leads to anaemia and chronic fatigue. The standard treatment for spherocytosis is to remove the spleen. In 2009, the most successful German Winter Olympian of all time, speed skater Claudia Pechstein, was given a two-year ban due to an accusation of blood doping. Her irregular levels of red blood cells were considered suspicious. Even though she produced evidence suggesting she inherited it from her father, the ban remained. After the ban was lifted, she returned to win Bronze in the 2011 World Championships.

Red blood cells are able to carry oxygen using haemoglobin, a complex molecule composed of globin proteins, and haem groups whose iron molecules temporarily link to oxygen. Mutations in the production of haem lead to a group of diseases called porphyria, while defects in globin cause thalassaemia.

Thalassaemias result from mutations causing reductions in either the alpha- or beta-globin proteins making up haemoglobin. Unlike most genes, there are two genes for alpha-globin on each chromosome: the more of these genes that are mutated, the more severe the disease. Defects in all four genes result in early death; three affected genes lead to the development of anaemia in childhood while two can cause mild anaemia. If only one of the four alpha genes is mutated then no symptoms are usually seen. There is only one gene for beta-globin. Inheriting two mutant copies leads to severe anaemia, called beta-thalassemia

161

major, which, if left untreated, results in death before the age of twenty. Inheriting only one mutant beta-globin gene leads to beta-thalassemia minor; a mild anaemia with some symptoms of fatigue, that are often unnoticed by the person.

The name thalassemia translates from Greek *thalassa* for the sea as it is most commonly found around areas of the Mediterranean in people of Italian Greek or North African descent. The reason, as in the case of sickle cell anaemia, is that carriers of

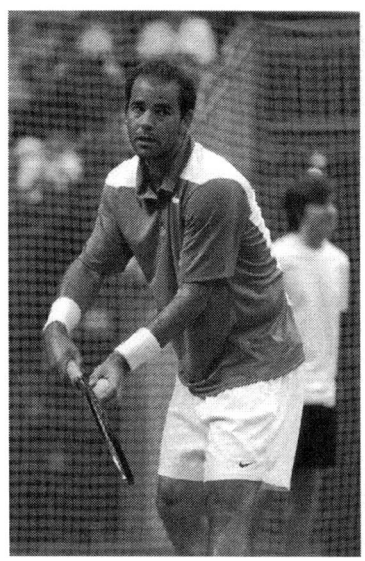

Pete Sampras

thalassemia mutations have a degree of protection against malaria. Pete Sampras, the son of Greek immigrants, has thalassemia minor, the symptoms of which sometimes troubled him during long hot-weather matches. After the Corretja match in the 1996 U.S. Open, a newspaper reported that he had Thalassemia. However, he did not admit it until he had broken the Grand Slam record in Wimbledon 2000 as he didn't want opponents to realise he was playing with a handicap.

Red blood cells rely on glucose as a source of energy through a biochemical pathway using the enzyme Glucose-6-phosphate dehydrogenase (G6PD) among others. Deficiency of this enzyme is the most common inherited enzyme deficiency disease in the world and results in an anaemic response to certain foods and chemicals such fava beans, also known as broad beans, and the antimalarial drug, primaquine. This is because G6PD also plays a role in protecting red blood cells against oxidative damage – fava beans contain extremely high amounts of oxidants which can damage G6PD-deficient cells.

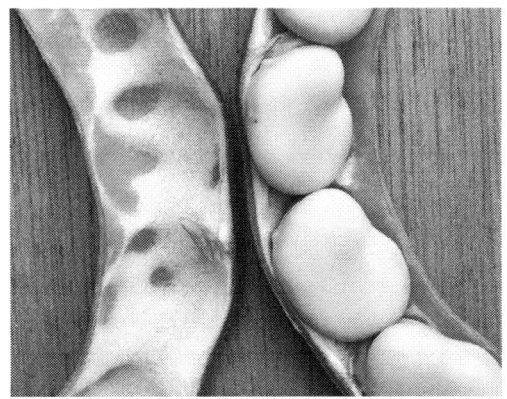

Broad beans, also known as fava beans

G6PD deficiency is possibly the first example of a pharmacogenetic disorder to be described, i.e. inherit differences in individual's sensitivity to particular chemicals. Pythagoras, around 500 BC in southern Italy, recognised that some individuals who ate fava beans became ill, suffering from symptoms of anaemia including jaundice and fatigue, while others could enjoy them with no adverse effects. This leads to the commonly used term "favism" for this disease and Pythagoras used to call on his disciples to abstain from beans. However, this has also been interpreted as Pythagoras advising his followers to stay away from politics; in ancient Greece and Rome, beans were used as a method of casting votes. Alternatively, he may have observed that the high sugar content of beans leads to flatulence! By the late 1940s, it was realised that the British, in contrast to Mediterranean populations, rarely developed haemolytic anaemia (increased destruction of blood cells) on ingestion of fava beans, suggesting a genetic cause. This became even more evident during the Korean War when around 10% of male American soldiers of African or Mediterranean-descent developed haemolytic anaemia in response to the antimalarial drug, primaquine, which was later discovered to be also due to G6PD deficiency. This was dramatized in an episode of *M*A*S*H** in which *Cpl Maxwell Klinger* exhibited all the symptoms of malaria but did not have the parasite. However, when he stopped taking primaquine, he recovered completely.

The reason G6PD deficiency is particularly prevalent in people of Mediterranean-descent – affecting as many as 1 in 10 – appears again to be due to the protective effect this condition has against malaria. The malaria-causing parasite, plasmodium, requires G6PD for its survival and replication in red blood cells. Since the mortality rate for favism is low and the mortality rate for malaria is high, the protective effect of the enzyme deficiency is significant. There are some villages in Sardinia where up to 70% are found to be G6PD deficient. Interestingly, this deficiency has also been connected to longevity. In centenarians, the incidence of G6PD deficiency is, on average, double compared to control groups. Some epidemiological studies have even suggested that G6PD deficiency may decrease susceptibility to cancer, cardiovascular disease and stroke.

Haemoglobin is composed of globin proteins combined with a molecule called haem. This consists of an organic ring structure called a porphyrin and an iron atom which is able to bind oxygen. In addition to its role in haemoglobin, haem also has other functions serving as a component of several liver enzymes. There are 8 steps involved in the making of haem from the 2 molecules glycine and succinyl-CoA, and each step is performed by a specific enzyme coded for by a different gene. If one of the different haem precursor molecules, known as porphyrins, is not modified, it cannot proceed to the next step and instead accumulates. The diseases caused by partial defects in these enzymes - a complete absence of haem production is not compatible with life - are known as porphyria (Gr. *porphyros*; purple). The name derives from the purple-red colour of the urine when the porphyrins are excreted. Affecting around 1 in 20,000 individuals, these porphyrins can accumulate in other parts of the body resulting in different physical and neurological symptoms, dependent upon which enzyme is affected and which porphyrin accumulates as a result.

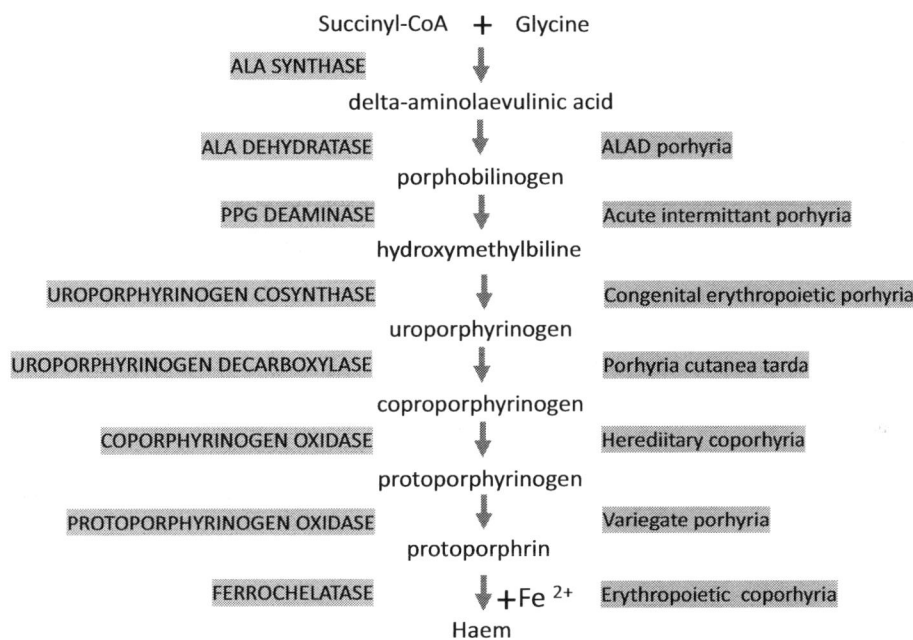

The pathway for heme production with specific enzymes (left) that when disrupted lead to diseases (right)

Acute intermittent porphyria results in the accumulation of specific porphyrins that are neurotoxins that lead to abdominal pain, tremors, seizures and also psychoses, including agitation and hallucinations, which can last for weeks and then quickly abate.

Though most people who inherit this trait do not develop the symptoms, precipitating factors for such attacks include hormones, drugs and alcohol that induce the production of haem in the liver. It has been suggested that Vincent van Gogh might have suffered from this disorder, leading to bouts of severe psychosis, which often involved suicide attempts and self-mutilation. Factors triggering his symptoms could have included overwork, fasting, malnutrition, and of course his famous absinthe binges. This might explain why, during his periods of hospitalisation, his symptoms abated with improved diet and lack of alcohol.

Defects in the fourth step of the haem pathway lead to congenital erythropoietic porphyria, also known as Gunther's disease. Here, a different porphyrin, that reacts to light, builds up causing severe skin blistering and photosensitivity. Sufferers tend to avoid daylight, show photosensitivity of eyes, develop a reddish fluorescing teeth enamel as the porphyrin collects there, a stretching of the lips causing teeth to become more prominent, an overgrowth of velus hair on the face, and muscle weakness especially in the wrists and fingers. Interestingly, garlic stimulates haem production and so can turn a mild case of porphyria into a very painful one. It has even been suggested that people suffering from

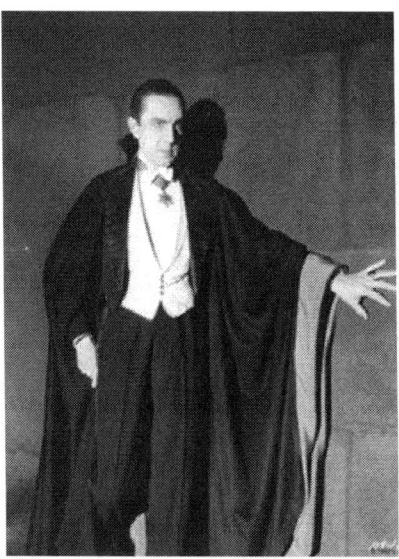

Lugosi as *Count Dracula* in the 1931 film

porphyria in past centuries might have been prescribed blood to drink in the mistaken belief that this could reduce the anaemia, which it certainly does not. Furthermore, although porphyrias are rare, it is believed to have been more common among Eastern European aristocracy, which was characterised by a high incidence of intermarriage. Many have suggested that cases of this disease in the past could have formed the basis of vampire legends. It is further recorded that Bram Stoker, before writing *Dracula*, met a psychiatric patient who exhibited symptoms including photosensitivity that could have helped to inspire his novel.

King George III, between 1788 and 1804, suffered bouts of "madness" involving a rapid pulse, fever, abdominal pains, constipation, cramp, skin blistering, *"port-wine-coloured"* urine, and rambling speech degenerating into obscenities and hallucinations. Just as each episode was acute in onset, the recovery phase was equally sudden and rapid. It has been suggested he may have suffered from a form of porphyria known as Variegata, caused by mutations in the gene for another enzyme in the haem production pathway. The term variegate describes the variable nature of the symptoms as most people do not experience any symptoms while others show a similar condition to that seen in acute intermittent

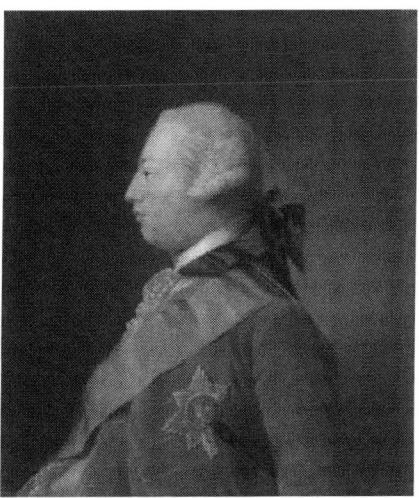

George III by Allan Ramsay, 1762

porphyria. It is possible this disease might be traced back to his ancestors, Mary Queen of Scots in the 1500s, and her son, King James I, whose physician noted urine "*red, like Alicante wine*". Other notable royal sufferers have been suggested to include James I's son Henry, Prince of Wales who had a similar illness and died suddenly, with allegations that he had been poisoned, the Duchess of Orleans who died of a sudden episode of excruciating abdominal pain, Queen Anne, George IV, and Princess Charlotte. Prince William of Gloucester, the grandson of George V, had reportedly been clinically diagnosed with porphyria, before dying in a plane crash aged 30, suggesting the presence of a gene defect in the family.

Erythropoietic protoporphyria (Gr. *protos*; first), which is due to a reduced level of the enzyme involved in the last step of the pathway converting protoporphyrin IX into haem, leads to extremely severe photosensitivity, with affected infants screaming soon after being taken out into the sun with exposure inducing second degree burns and scarring of the skin seen in adulthood. It has been loosely suggested that a builder involved in the construction of the Paris Opera house, who lived in its cellar, perhaps to avoid sunlight, may have inspired the French writer Gaston Leroux to create *The Phantom of the Opera*.

The average person's body contains around 5 litres of blood, which is composed of about 60% liquid plasma, made up mainly of water, and 40% cells. All the different types of blood cells are manufactured from stem cells found in the bone marrow. These stem cells divide and form into red blood cells called erythrocytes (Gr. *erythros*; red), white blood cells known as leukocytes (Gr. *leuko*; white), and platelets which are also known as thrombocytes (Gr. *thrombo*; clotting). Diseases resulting in a disruption of bone marrow can lead to reduced numbers of blood cells, such as found in the disorder Fanconi anaemia. Some conditions, such as polycythaemia (Lat. *poly*; many, *cyt*; cell, *haemia*; blood), can lead to the bone marrow being stimulated to increase the production of blood cells.

Some mutations can result in increased red blood cell numbers. One such mutation increases the efficiency of a hormone secreted from the kidneys, called erythropoietin (EPO), to stimulate the bone marrow to produce more red blood cells. The increased numbers of these red blood cells and the corresponding increase in oxygen levels in the blood can lead to greater athleticism and endurance. For example, the cross-country skier Eero Mäntyranta, one of Finland's most successful skiers was shown to have had hereditary polycythaemia following a DNA study on over 200 members of his family. However, this defect and other disorders resulting in increased numbers of red blood cells, can lead to capillaries becoming clogged by the increased viscosity of the blood. As a result, untreated sufferers are at risk of thrombosis, heart attacks and strokes.

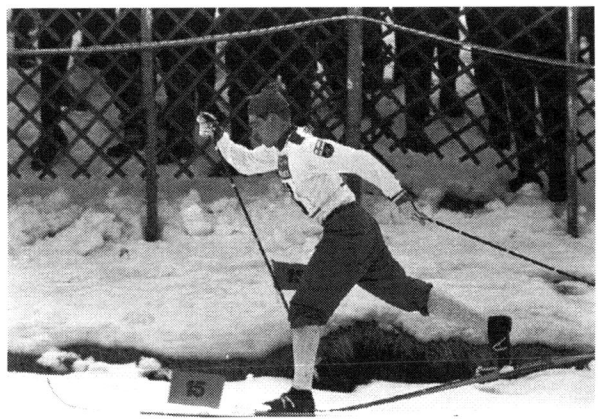

Eero Mäntyranta, Innsbruck olympic games 1964

As a treatment for anaemia, drugs have been developed that mimic the EPO hormone in order to stimulate red blood cell production. However, some sportsmen realised that the EPO drugs could help their blood to carry more oxygen and so allow their bodies to work harder for longer. Consequently, by the late 1990s, EPO-abuse had rocketed with athletes seemingly blind to the dangers associated with increased blood hyper-viscosity. For example, this has been linked to the deaths of 18 Dutch and Belgian cyclists between 1987 and 1990; it may also have contributed to a number of Tour de France wins. Despite the medical and professional risks EPO abuse still remains rife in many professional sports.

Red blood cells are produced from stem cells in the red bone marrow of our long bones. Diseases impairing the ability of bone marrow to produce enough new blood cells can lead to anaemia. One example is Fanconi anaemia, named after the Swiss paediatrician Guido Fanconi who described a family in 1927 with 3 affected children. Genes coding for DNA repair become mutated slowing down the ability of cells to overcome and repair DNA damage. This leads to reduced production of blood cells and anaemia, an increased risk of leukaemia as cells are less able to repair damaged DNA, susceptibility to infection, fatigue and haemorrhaging.

Parents of a girl called Molly Nash, born with Fanconi anaemia, embarked upon a controversial procedure to conceive another child who could provide bone marrow to help cure their daughter. In the year 2000, they underwent in vitro fertilisation, known as IVF, where egg cells are fertilised outside of a woman's body and grown to the 6 or 8 cell stage and then transferred back to the mother. However, in the Nash's case the embryos were genetically tested for signs of the Fanconi anaemia-causing gene and only an embryo that did not carry the genetic abnormality, and therefore a safe donor match for Molly, was then implanted into her mother. Following this procedure, a healthy boy named Adam was born. Dubbed *"Little Frankenstein"* by the New York Post in 2000, blood from his umbilical cord containing stem cells was infused into his sister. The procedure sparked much debate and criticism from various individuals. But importantly, both children are still fine, and

Molly is now able to lead a relatively normal life.

Blood clotting, for example following a cut in the skin, is accomplished by a complicated process involving many different proteins in the blood called clotting factors together with platelet cells. Inherited defects in these clotting factors can lead to increased bleeding seen in haemophilia. Disruption of platelets can lead to increased blood clotting found in disorders such as thrombocytopenia or von Willebrand's disease.

Individuals with haemophilia can bleed for prolonged times lasting for days, and even weeks, in response to relatively minor injuries. This disorder mostly affects males as the genes for the two major affected blood clotting factors, factor VIII (resulting in haemophilia A) and factor IX (haemophilia B), are both located on the X chromosome. First acquiring the name of haemophilia from a Swiss doctor in 1828, this could be one of the earliest recognised inherited illnesses. Well over 2,000 years ago, Jewish rabbis referred to a bleeding condition that was fatal to young boys and ran in families, drawing up guidelines to exempt males from circumcision if they had brothers who had previously died from the procedure.

The British royal family has included many males with haemophilia in addition to female carriers including Queen Victoria herself. Recent genetic analysis has shown this to be haemophilia B. Queen Victoria seems to have spontaneously acquired the haemophilia mutation de nova, as her parents' families are not known to have had the disease. However, her paternity has been questioned! She then passed on this mutated clotting factor IX gene to her son Prince Leopold, Duke of Albany and, through several of her daughters, to various royal houses across the continent such as the Spanish, German and Russian royal families. Prince Leopold, finding that his joint pain, which was another symptom of his haemophilia, was aggravated by cold weather, would seek warmer climates abroad during the winter. And it was while in the south of France, in March 1884, that he slipped and fell in the Yacht Club in Cannes, injuring his knee and dying the next morning. His only daughter, Princess Alice of Albany, then passed the gene on to her oldest son, Prince Rupert of Teck, who bled to death after a car accident at the age of 20. Queen Victoria's granddaughter, Czarina Alexandra of Russia, passed the disease on to her son Alexei. Desperate to cure their son the Russian royal family turned to the 'mad monk' Rasputin whose influence over the family is often cited as a main catalyst for the Russian revolution. His treatment involved hypnosis, a calming confident presence around the boy and family, and exclusion of all the other court physicians who may have been stressful for the young Alexia. It is now known that hypnosis and reduction of stress narrows minor arteries slowing blood circulation and so relieving symptoms. Although it seems unlikely that Rasputin was aware of this, his pervading influence over the royal household played a part in their eventual executions.

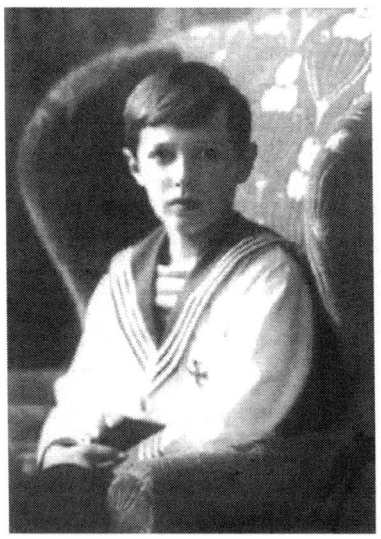

Alexei Nicholaevitch Romanov, 1913

It was only following the development of blood transfusion, that treatment involving the infusion of blood clotting factors became available increasing life expectancy considerably. However, in the UK, contaminated blood led to the widespread infection of HIV and Hepatitis C in haemophiliacs. Heat and chemical treatment of blood products were introduced in 1986 to eliminate such viruses, and since 1992 'recombinant' clotting factors, produced by genetic engineering, are now used. Unfortunately, there is still no permanent way of replacing or enabling the body to synthesise a functional clotting factor.

Von Willebrand factor, named after Finnish the physician, who first described it in the 1920s, is a protein involved in controlling the activity of platelet cells important in blood clotting. Mutations in the gene coding for this protein leads to the most common hereditary coagulation disorder, von Willebrand's disease. Three different types of von Willebrand's disease exist differing in severity, from the rare severe form to the relatively common mild forms characterised by only slightly prolonged bleeding, possibly affecting as many as 1 per cent of the population. These mild forms can be a complication in child abuse cases, as it can cause children to bruise easily. One person who suffered from the severe type of von Willebrand disease was the musician Bill Kozlowski, founder of the Alaskan rock band *Peabody's Monster*. Much of Kozlowski's song-writing focuses on living life to the fullest, as he knew his lifespan would be limited. He would suffer internal bleeds that often left him in severe pain and cartilage deterioration that resulted in numerous surgeries on his legs. He died at 32 years of age from a heart attack.

When blood vessels are damaged, collagen becomes exposed, causing platelet cells to aggregate through binding via a receptor protein found on their cell surface. Mutations in the gene for this receptor can lead to reduced platelet adhesion and prolonged lengths of bleeding, a condition known as Glanzmann's thrombasthenia (Gr. *thromb*, lump/blood clot;

asthenia, weakness). Another very common mutation in a gene for the receptor, carried by about 20 per cent of the population, can predispose individuals to a higher risk of developing acute coronary artery events. On November 20th 1995, the Russian two-times Olympic Gold medallist and four-time world champion skater, Sergei Grinkov, died suddenly of a massive heart attack, while in the middle of a practice session. He was only 28 years old and, though having none of the typical risk factors associated with heart disease, his autopsy revealed he had severe coronary artery disease with a subsequent DNA test revealing he had the causal gene variation.

Thrombotic diseases are characterised by the formation of a thrombus, or blood clot, which can obstruct blood flow. It is suggested that, of all the patients suffering from thromboembolisms, over a quarter have some genetic predisposition. For example, around 5 per cent of Caucasians have a polymorphism in the factor V gene, known as the Factor V Leiden mutation after the place it was discovered, which causes an increase in blood clotting. Inheriting one copy of the mutation increases between 4 to 8-fold the chance of developing a clot while those with two copies of the mutation may have up to 80 times the usual risk of developing a blood clot. Though there is no cure, identifying a genetic risk allows treatment, which can include lifelong prescription with an anticoagulant such as warfarin which inhibits the production of some of these clotting factors. Initially, warfarin was developed as a rat poison, but it was not until a sailor in the US Navy tried, unsuccessfully, to commit suicide in 1951 by drinking it, that its use as a therapeutic anticoagulant was considered. Interestingly, warfarin was used to treat one world leader, Dwight Eisenhower after his heart attack in 1955, and possibly used to dispatch another, Joseph Stalin, in 1953.

Some people are born with blood vessels that have not developed properly. In Hereditary haemorrhagic telangiectasia, these abnormal blood vessels, known as telangiectasia, may appear just underneath the skin, which shows as red or purple spots. This disorder can cause frequent bleeding, anaemia, seizures and increased risks of stroke. Generally inherited autosomal dominantly, it is thought to be caused by mutations in genes

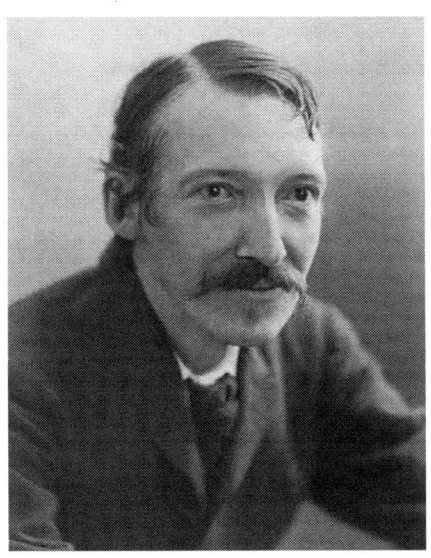

Robert Louis Stevenson, 1893

important for producing proteins found in the lining of the blood vessels. It has been suggested that the famed Scottish author Robert Louis Stevenson may have suffered from this disease, explaining his chronic respiratory problems, bleeding in the lungs, and his death, at age 44 years, following a probable stroke. That his mother also died from an apparent stroke, at the relatively young age of 38 years old, may support inheritance of the condition.

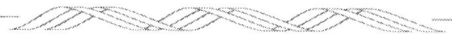

# IMMUNE DISORDERS

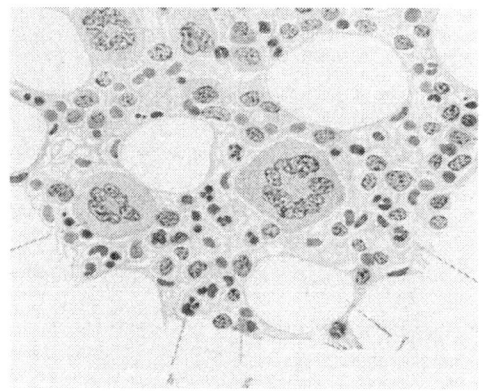

*Sick of hearing this shit about me not talking... not true... good days, bad days... but I still am a talkin'*
*motherfucker!*

Richard Pryor, post on rebutting reports he had lost his voice.

The immune system describes the collection of biological processes within our body that
serves to protect us against disease by identifying and killing pathogens. We have a special
type of immune response known as the adaptive immune response; 'adaptive' in that it is

176

able to recognise and remember specific pathogens to generate an immune memory, known as immunity. This allows our bodies to mount stronger attacks each time a pathogen is next encountered. As part of the immune system, we have phagocyte (Gr. *phago*, eat) cells in the blood that are able to engulf foreign cells and proteins. Defects in these cells can lead to chronic granulomatous disease. Other cells found in the blood, known as T-lymphocytes (T-cells) are able to recognise foreign proteins, known as antigens, and release chemicals to further break down this foreign material and attract and stimulate the division of further immune cells. These antigens are also bound by another type of immune cell, B-lymphocytes (B-cells), causing these cells to divide and produce antibodies (immunoglobulins; Ig). Antibodies then function to destroy antigens, such as on invading pathogens, by causing them to precipitate or clump and can, in addition, initiate further pathways that cause the destruction of the antigen and stop the antigen from entering host cells. Some of the activated B cells and T cells can go on to become memory cells that divide and reproduce extremely quickly following exposure to the same invading pathogenic antigen, such as a flu virus for example, at any point later in the individual's lifetime. Defects in this system lead to severe combined immunodeficiency syndrome.

Perhaps the earliest documented incidence of acquired immunity was during the

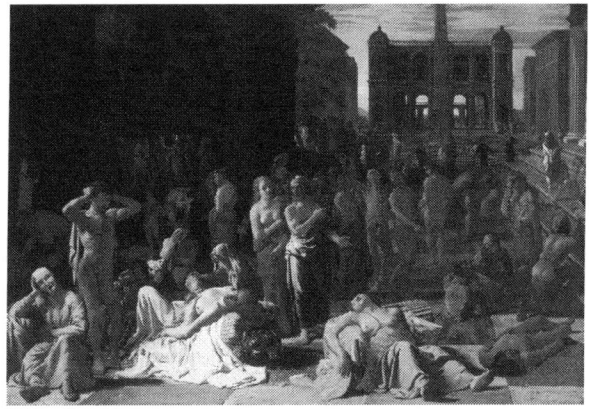

*The Plague of Athens* by Michael Sweerts, 1652

177

plague of Athens in 430 BC. Here it was noted at the time that people who had recovered from a previous bout of the disease could nurse the sick without contracting the illness a second time. This forms the basis of vaccination whereby a substance is introduced into the body in order to produce immunity to a disease.

Although similar procedures may have been used in China and India in ancient times, the first recorded vaccination, was by Edward Jenner in 1796. He used puss from cowpox blisters to give people immunity against the very similar pathogen smallpox, after observing that dairymaids who had previously been sick with cowpox, contracted from infected cow's udders, did not catch smallpox. Vaccine derives from the Latin *vacca* for cow. Pasteur then further developed the use of artificial vaccines that could be used for a variety of diseases such as rabies by growing the virus in dogs and rabbits, then destroying the virus by drying the affected tissues, and then reintroducing it into healthy animals. This serves to activate an immune response against parts of a dead virus to form an immune memory so that when coming into contact with the infectious form of the virus the immune system can quickly respond.

Before the advent of antibiotic drugs, most babies born with inherited immune defects would have died early due to their susceptibility to infections and such cases would not have been easy to identify among the many immunologically normal infants who would have also died of infections. It was not until 1952 that the first immunodeficiency disease was described, by Dr Colonel Ogden Bruton, when he reported the failure of a male child to produce antibodies due to a defective gene hindering B-cell growth. This is now known as Bruton's X-linked agammaglobulinemia, as the gene involved is found on the X chromosome. Dr Bruton also became the first physician to provide specific immunotherapy for this disorder by administering injections of antibodies to the patient who responded well to the treatment. Since then, many more diseases of antibody production have been described, where affected infants usually develop recurrent infections with pyogenic, or pus-forming, bacteria such as pneumonia-causing *Streptococcus pneumoniae*.

The most common inherited immunodeficiency is selective IgA antibody deficiency, present in around 1 in 400 people. While it seems to result in no specific symptoms it is found more often in people with chronic lung disease. Aside from IgA deficiency, the overall incidence of primary immunodeficiency is around 1 in 10,000.

Patients with defects in T-cell development are highly susceptible to a broad range of infectious agents, highlighting the importance of T-cells in many parts of the immune system. Such diseases are known as Severe Combined Immunodeficiency (SCID) as patients are unable to generate any immune memory. Consequently, they suffer infections from many opportunistic pathogens that can lead to early death if untreated. Treatment can include transplantations of bone marrow that enable the production of T-cells and B-cells. The most common type of SCID is called XSCID due to the mutated gene being found on the X chromosome. This gene normally codes for part of a protein receptor on the surface of T-cells allowing them to develop properly and from immunological memories.

Awareness of these diseases was raised in the 1970s by the plight of David Vetter, who lived nearly all of his 12 years of life inside a sealed plastic bubble designed to protect him from infections. David Vetter's parents first had a daughter, Katherine, who was healthy and then a son who died six months after birth from SCID. They realised that any subsequent child would have a 50 per cent chance of inheriting the same condition but believing that a bone marrow transplant from their healthy daughter would give any

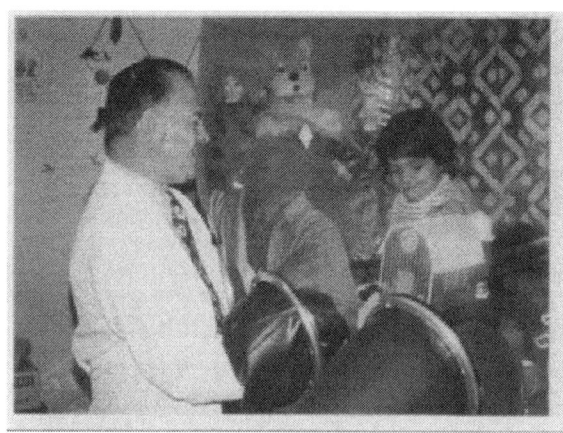

David Vetter, *circa* 1978

infected child a normal healthy life, they decided to go through with another pregnancy. Twenty seconds after being removed from his mother's womb, in September 1971, David Vetter was sealed in a germ-free environment that would be his home for almost his entire life. Water, air, food, diapers and clothes were all disinfected with special cleaning agents before entering his cocoon and he was handled only through special plastic gloves attached to the walls. Eventually, a bone marrow transplant was performed using marrow donated by his sister Katherine. However, a few months after the operation, David started having diarrhoea, fever and severe vomiting, requiring him to be taken out of his sealed contained for the first time in 1984, for treatment. However, he died 15 days later of a lymphoma, caused by an unscreened virus, in his newly transplanted bone marrow.

Phagocytic cells destroy foreign matter, such as microorganisms by ingesting them into their cells where various enzymes break them down. There are a number of gene mutations that can lead to defects in the ability of phagocytes cells to kill pathogens. This occurs in chronic granulomatous disease due to mutations in a number of different genes, leading to recurrent bacterial infections.

While deficiencies in the immune system can lead to infections, an overactive immune system can lead to another class of diseases known as autoimmune diseases. These are characterised by a decreased ability of the immune system to distinguish between foreign material and the persons own cells and tissues. As a result, an individual's immune system attacks its own tissues. There are more than forty different autoimmune diseases affecting around 5 to 10 per cent of the population with women accounting for around three-quarters of all cases.

Some people are born with an inherited genetic susceptibility to autoimmune diseases. Such genetic risk factors often involve the inheritance of specific variants of genes called Human Lymphocyte Antigens (HLA). These HLA proteins are produced and displayed on the outside of all the cells in our bodies and function by presenting fragments of all the types of proteins contained within the cell, on the outside of the cells. This will include host cell proteins or proteins from any possible invading pathogens. T-cells that recognise a protein from a pathogen then assume the cell is infected and destroy the cell. If the T-cell wrongly considers a host protein as a pathogen, it will kill all those healthy cells that produce that protein. Depending upon which proteins are recognised, different cells may be subsequently attacked and a number of different diseases can develop. For example, an immune reaction against cells of the thyroid gland can lead to altered thyroid hormone production seen in Grave's disease. President George H. W. Bush was diagnosed in 1991 shortly after his wife Barbara and their dog Millie, purely by chance. However, because of the remarkable coincidence that all three cases of an autoimmune disease occurred in one household, it was once suspected that this may have been the result of a plot to poison the President. The Secret Service went as far as to test the water in all of the presidential residences, including the White House, for any toxins. Many pictures of Barbara Bush during this period show that she had developed many of the classical characteristics of the disease, such as a bulging of the eyes and a throat goitre. The wife of Vladimir Lenin,

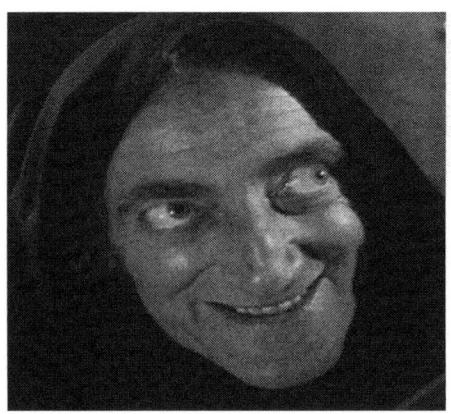

Marty Feldman as *Igor* in *Young Frankenstein*, 1974

Nadezhda Krupskaya, may also have suffered from Graves's disease - her bulging eyes giving her the Bolshevik codename of *Fish*. Since Graves' Disease can also disrupt the menstrual cycle, it is a possible explanation as to why the couple never had children. The British comedian Marty Feldman incorporated the bulging eyes from his Graves's disease into many of his comedy routines.

The body may also start to produce an immune response antibody against specific proteins known as neurotransmitters in the disease Myasthenia Gravis. This has the effect of blocking nerve signals to muscle cells resulting in muscle weakness. Suzanne Rogers, an American actress best known for her role in the daytime television series *Days of Our Lives*, was diagnosed with Myasthenia Gravis in 1984 and insisted that her character, *Maggie*, be diagnosed with the same disease on the show in order to raise awareness of the condition. In another neurological disorder, the immune system attacks the myelin sheath surrounding nerve cell axons. This is known as multiple sclerosis. It is generally believed that it results from an early infection which primes a susceptible immune system to mistakenly recognise and destroy myelin later in life. The body then tries to repair the damage with hard plaques of scar tissue, known as sclerosis, which further disrupts the flow of electrical impulses between nerve cells. Although not considered a hereditary disease, genetics does play some role in determining susceptibility. For example, in studies of identical twins, the likelihood that the second twin may develop multiple sclerosis if the first twin does is about 30 per cent.

One of the earliest people to be diagnosed with multiple sclerosis was Sir Augustus Frederick d'Este, grandson of George III. He left a highly detailed diary describing his 22 years living with the disease. His symptoms began at the age of 28 with weakness of his legs, clumsiness of the hands, numbness, dizziness and bladder disturbances that worsened until 1844 when he was confined to a wheelchair and dying shortly after. The American comedian, Richard Pryor, in his later years became a wheelchair user due to MS, which he said stood for *"More Shit"*. He was diagnosed in 1986, after experiencing slight disorientation, but went on to develop drifting eyes, vertigo, tremors, muscle weakness, prickling sensations in the skin and chronic fatigue. In 1995, he played an embittered multiple sclerosis patient in an episode of the television series *Chicago Hope*, which earned him an Emmy nomination. He died in 2005 aged 65 of a heart attack.

While some autoimmune diseases occur due to an immune response to a specific cell or tissue, others are characterised by general tissue damage throughout the body. This is seen in systemic lupus erythematosus where antibodies are produced that bind to cells in many tissues of the body causing the immune system to attack and damage various parts of the body including the joints, skin, kidneys, heart lungs, blood vessels and brain. Possibly first described by Hippocrates in the year 400 BC, the term lupus is attributed to the 12th-century physician Rogerius, who used it to describe the classic reddish, butterfly-shaped rash across the nose and cheeks – the name either deriving from the Latin for wolf as it can resemble the pattern of fur on a wolf's face or from a French style of mask which women reportedly wore to conceal the characteristic rash on their faces. Systemic lupus erythematosus has some genetic link and can run in families, with several genes identified, however, symptoms and severity vary enormously between individuals. There are two main types of lupus. One form, discoid lupus, only affects the skin. Systemic lupus erythematosus, however, harms the skin, joints, kidneys and brain. The English singer/songwriter, Seal, was diagnosed with the skin-affecting variant of this condition as a young man which has left him with the distinctive facial scars on his cheeks. Other singers have battled the systemic condition. In 2015, Selena Gomez revealed she had been diagnosed with a severe form of systemic lupus erythematosus, that required chemotherapy and then a kidney transplant, donated by her long-time friend, the actress Francia Raisa. Lady Gaga has spoken about being borderline positive for the disease and has several relatives with the condition. She also suffers chronically from fibromyalgia, that shares many symptoms with lupus and can occur together with it. This chronic condition of widespread pain and profound fatigue was the reason behind her having to cancel her 2017 European tour. She has since made a Netflix documentary, *Gaga: Five Foot Two*, to raise awareness of the condition.

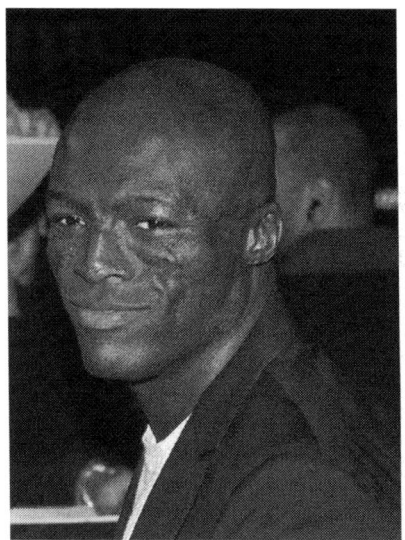

Seal, 2008

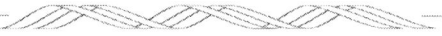

# ENDOCRINE DISORDERS

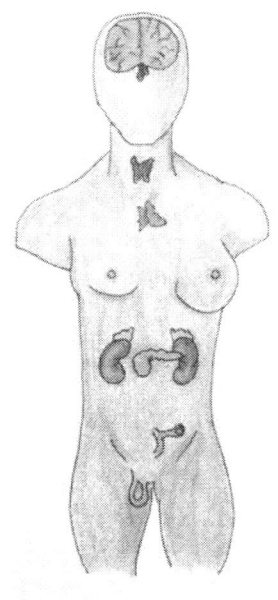

*Diabetes has to live with me, rather than me live with diabetes*

Steven Redgrave

Our endocrine system comprises a group of glands and organs that regulate and control various body functions by releasing specific proteins or steroids known as hormones. These are released into the bloodstream where they act as messengers, affecting the various activities of different tissues and organs. Each type of hormone influences only certain organs and tissues. When a particular hormone reaches its target cell it transmits its message by binding to a receptor, on the cell surface or in the cell, causing the cell to take a specific action. In this way, very small amounts of hormones can trigger very large responses in the body affecting such diverse processes as growth and development, reproduction, metabolism and sexual characteristics.

The endocrine system includes the hypothalamus, the pituitary, pineal, thyroid, parathyroid, thymus, pancreas, adrenals, testes and the ovaries. There are also numerous other organs and tissues that also have endocrine functions such as the stomach and heart. It is important that the levels of hormones are regulated within precise limits; to do this, many endocrine glands are controlled by an interplay of hormonal signals between the hypothalamus, located in the brain, and the pituitary gland, which sits at the base of the brain.

The hypothalamus is a region of the brain that secretes a number of hormones known as releasing hormones, as these further stimulate the secretion of hormones from the

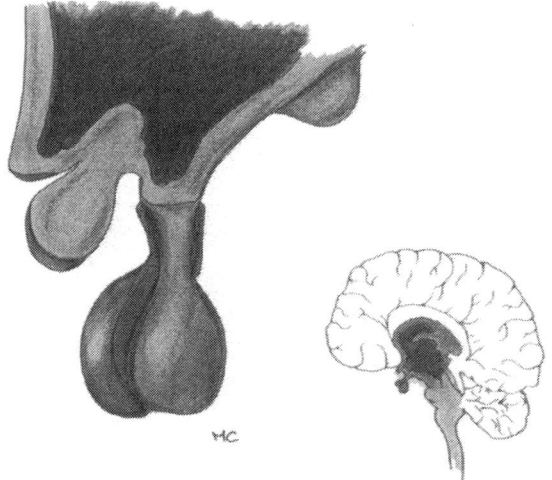

Hypothalamus and pituitary gland

pituitary gland. For example, gonadotropin-releasing hormone released from the hypothalamus signals the pituitary to produce follicle-stimulating hormone and luteinising hormone which, in turn, stimulate the ovaries or testes to produce yet further hormones, such as testosterone and oestrogen, to signal sexual development. An inherited deficiency of gonadotropin-releasing hormone, therefore, results in the absence or decreased function of testes or ovaries. This is known as Kallmann syndrome. First described in 1944 by the German geneticist, Franz Josef Kallmann, this syndrome generally presents with hypogonadism (i.e. an underproduction of testosterone), delayed puberty and a lack of secondary sex characteristics. Jimmy Scott, the famed American jazz and blues vocalist, had very short stature and an unusually high-pitched voice, which never broke, due to the effects of this syndrome delaying puberty. However, he married five times, having one son, before dying in 2014 aged 88.

Two further hypothalamic hormones are vasopressin and oxytocin that are released through the pituitary. A main job of vasopressin is to maintain water balance by regulating levels of water excreted by the kidneys. A lack of vasopressin leads to large amounts of water being excreted by the kidneys – a condition known as diabetes insipidus (Gr. *diabainein*, to stand with legs apart, implying urination; *insipidus*, without taste implying very dilute). A person with diabetes insipidus can urinate as much as 18 litres daily – the average urine volume for a normal adult is 1.5 litres – which is naturally also accompanied by excessive thirst. It was only in 1792 that this genetic disorder was first described in the medical literature through a study of a French woman who drank over 20 litres of water a day. Since the age of 3, she had remembered drinking buckets of water, until, in her early teens when she was forced out of home by her probably bewildered, parents. This disease is usually caused by mutations in the gene for vasopressin that regulates levels of water excreted by the kidneys.

There is a very old Scottish tale of a gipsy woman travelling with her thirsty son who was denied water by a housewife. The gipsy woman then cursed the housewife, causing the housewife's sons to crave water while condemning her daughters to pass the curse on to future generations. This is a description of a far rarer form of diabetes insipidus resulting from mutations in a receptor for vasopressin found on the X chromosome, so leading to a sex-linked inherited from, specifically affecting males. Two Scotsmen immigrated with the mutant gene to Nova Scotia, Canada, in 1761 arriving on a ship named the *Hopewell*. As a result, this disease is relatively common in some regions of Canada. Considering that fresh-water supplies on board a ship would have been limited, the journey for the two Scottish immigrants must have been an incredible ordeal.

The pituitary (Lat. *pituita*; mucus, as this gland was once thought to produce nasal mucus) gland is a pea-sized structure located at the base of the brain. It secretes several hormones including growth hormone, adrenocorticotropic hormone, follicle-stimulating hormone, luteinizing hormone, prolactin, melanocyte-stimulating hormone, and endorphins that inhibit pain sensations and help control the immune system.

The pituitary constantly produces a regulated supply of growth hormone that, secreted into the bloodstream, stimulates cells of the body to grow and divide ensuring that all portions of the body grow at an equal rate. Increased production of growth hormone can occur as a result of a pituitary tumour. When this tumour develops during childhood a condition known as gigantism can occur characterised by lengthening bones, especially in the arms and legs, resulting in the individual growing to an unusually great height, often 7ft (213 cm) to 9ft tall (274 cm).

Perhaps the first written account of a giant comes from the bible, as Goliath was described as either four or six "cubits" which equals around 6ft 9in (206 cm) or 9ft 6in (320 cm). People afflicted with gigantism continue to grow throughout their lives. One well-known individual with gigantism, called Charles Byrne, had an enlarged pituitary comparable in size to a peach. Known as the *Irish Giant* he grew to a height of 7ft 9in (236 cm). His exceptional height generated great interest in various physicians who would

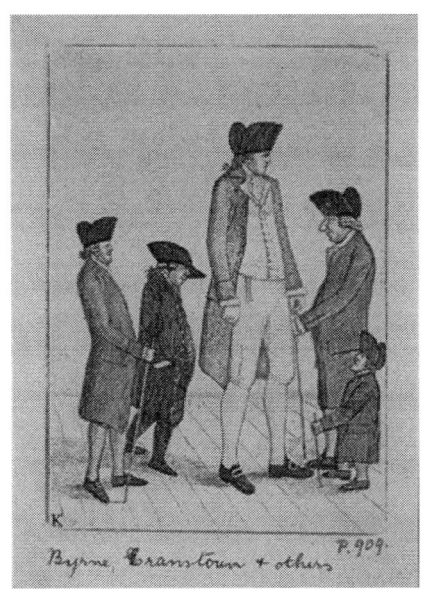

Charles Byrne, a person with short stature, and three average-sized men by J. Kay, 1794

constantly hound him in the hope of getting his body on their autopsy table. One in particular, John Hunter, supposedly would taunt him promising to boil his bones – a major fear that Charles Byrne had. It was supposedly this that drove Charles Byrne into drinking himself to death in 1783 at the age of 22. So afraid was he that John Hunter and the other doctors would get their hands on his body, Charles Byrne requested from his deathbed that he be buried at sea. However, John Hunter was quickly on the scene to bribe the hospital staff, purchasing the cadaver for 500 pounds. After boiling his bones in large copper kettle, his skeleton was put together, where it still resides in the Royal College of Surgeons. Recent analyses of DNA taken from Charles' teeth showed he had inherited a mutation for a gene important for the development of the pituitary and found in a number of living Irish families who are suffering from this hereditary disorder today. A literal interpretation of the Books of Samuel and Chronicles in the Bible states that Goliath had a brother and three sons with giant stature also suggestive of a hereditary gene for his disorder.

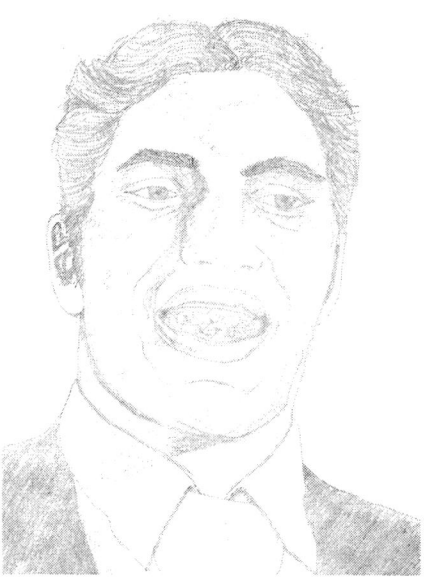

Richard Kiel

Acromegaly (Gr. *acro*; end, *mega*; large) occurs when too much growth hormone suddenly begins to be produced in adulthood, usually due to the development of a pituitary tumour. As this growth is signalled to occur long after the ends of the bones have hardened and cease to elongate, the bones rather than lengthening, become deformed. Often, the jawbone can overgrow and cartilage in the voice box can thicken, making the voice deep and husky. A major complication is joint pain and arthritis with some individuals also feeling weaknesses in their limbs, loss of vision and severe headaches as the enlarging tissues compress nerves. Film actors with this condition have inevitably been cast in intimidating roles such as 7ft 2in (217 cm) tall Richard Kiel who played *Jaws* in the *James Bond* movies, and also Ted Cassidy and Carel Stryken who both played the character *Lurch* in *The Addams Family*. An extreme example of how the disease can distort the skull and face can be seen in Rondo Hatton. Voted the most handsome boy at school, thirteen years later he was playing a contestant in an ugly man competition which he loses to a heavily made-up Charles Laughton as the *Hunchback of Notre Dame*. Achieving cult status for his roles in horror movies, it is sadly ironic that his only lead role was in his final movie *The Brute Man*, where he played a handsome college student scarred and turned into a monster by a chemical accident. He died only a few months after the move was finished in 1946 aged 51 years old from a heart attack linked to the disorder.

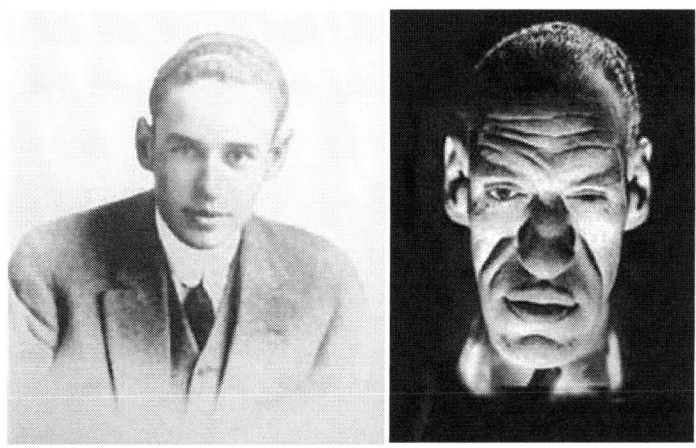

Rondo Hatton aged 19 and in his 40s

If the pituitary gland does not produce enough growth hormone in childhood, then an abnormally short stature may result, in which growth in all body parts are restricted to an equal degree. Count Josef Boruwlaski, born in Poland 1739 to averaged-sized parents, suffered from such a growth hormone deficit reaching a height of 2ft 4in (71 cm). That one

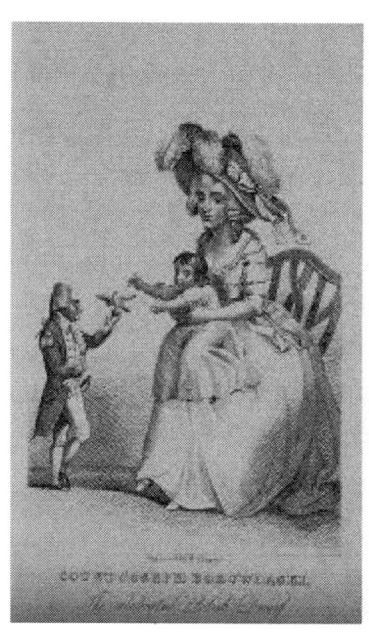

Joźef Boruwlaski, possibly with his wife and child

other of Josef's four siblings also showed severe height restriction, suggests that an inherited genetic defect may lay behind the condition. When he was 9 years old, a wealthy noblewoman, Staorina de Caorliz, took him to live with her to be educated and as a result, he entered into the highest levels of society, becoming favoured in Royal courts all over Europe. He married, fathering a child of normal body size, and moved to a village near Durham where he lived until his death in 1837, aged 98. It is thought that similar mutations affect pygmy tribes, a term which is sometimes applied to communities in which the height of individuals does not exceed 4ft 11in (150 cm). One such mutation found in the gene for growth hormone receptor occurs in a group of people living in the foothills of the Ecuadorian Andes. Known as Laron syndrome, there are around 350 people with it, who are descendants of a single ancestor who introduced the mutated gene thousands of years ago. These individuals don't lack growth hormone, but their defective receptor for this hormone means they are unable to react to the growth signals and consequently develop reduced height. However, the absence of this receptor is thought to reduce uncontrolled cell growth and increased sensitivity to insulin, so protecting these individuals against both the development of cancer and of diabetes. The incidence of heart disease and Alzheimer's

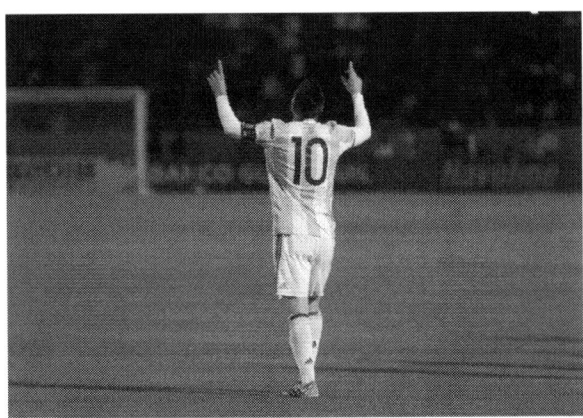

Lionel Messi, 2017

disease are also lower in these individuals. Like Joseph Boruwlaski, many of these individuals live to a relatively old age.

Growth hormone deficiency is now often treated with daily injections of growth hormone using a recombinant version of the hormone produced by genetically engineered bacteria. Lionel Messi, arguably one of the greatest football players in history, was diagnosed with growth hormone deficiency at the age of 11. Barcelona agreed, as part of his contract to sign him at the age of 12, to pay for all his medical treatment bills including the growth hormone treatments that he finished at the age of 14.

Another pituitary hormone, prolactin, is secreted in increased concentrations during pregnancy resulting in enlargement of the mammary glands and an increase in the production of milk. Around 30 per cent of pituitary tumours lead to a higher production of prolactin and increased lactation in women who are not pregnant. Accompanying the increased lactation is the suppression of ovulation as prolactin inhibits ovulation to stop further pregnancies occurring during breastfeeding. Known as hyperprolactinaemia, it is associated with phantom pregnancy syndrome with women visiting their gynaecologist thinking that they might be pregnant. It has been suggested that this disorder may have affected Queen Mary I of England. Married to Philip II of Spain she had two phantom pregnancies including swelling breasts and abdomen, discharges of milk, changes in appetite and mood and absolute conviction that she was carrying a child. However, this all

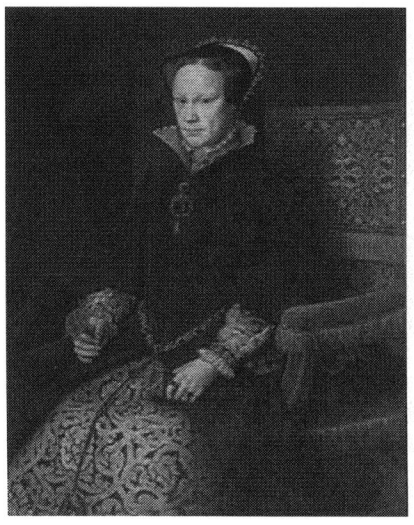

Mary I of England by Antonis Mor, 1554

ended in humiliation and political turmoil for Mary who died childless leaving her half-sister Elizabeth to succeed her.

The thyroid gland is situated to the front of the neck and is named after an ancient Greek army shield, known as "*thyreos*", which is shaped like a door with a notch at the top for the soldier's chin. This gland secretes the hormone thyroxine that controls metabolism, respiration, and heart function. Too little thyroxine is known

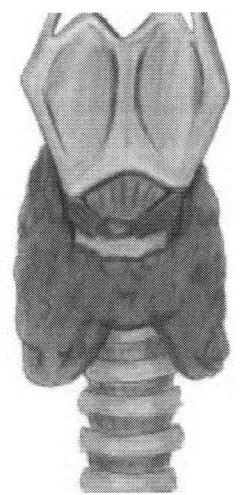

Thyroid gland

as hypothyroidism while diseases such as Grave's disease lead to increased hormone production, known as hyperthyroidism.

The majority of cases of hypothyroidism occur due to a lack of iodine in the diet required to make thyroid hormones. If this element is deficient in early childhood then growth can become stunted. An old, now offensive, term for this disease was cretinism; *Crétin* is an old French name for the wild men of the Alps in French folktales as this disease was for many centuries more common in areas where the soil is deficient in iodine – particularly in the Alpine regions of Europe. A further sign of this disease, particularly in adulthood, is enlarged thyroids, known as goitres, as the thyroid attempts to make up for the hormone reduction. This used to be common in the Carboniferous Limestone area of Derbyshire where soils are naturally low in iodine, and for this reason the condition was often referred to at the time as the "Derbyshire Neck". This problem was eventually tackled with the introduction of iodised milk, generally produced by increasing the iodine content of cattle feed.

Congenital hypothyroidism describes the presence of too little thyroxine production from birth. Affecting approximately 1 in 4,000 new-born infants, it's the most prevalent inborn endocrine disorder and can result from mutations in a number of different genes involved in thyroid hormone production. If not properly treated with daily doses of thyroid hormone, growth failure and permanent mental retardation can develop. The French actor Hervé Villechaize was born with a form of short-stature that related to thyroid dysfunction. Standing 3ft 11in (119 cm) tall he is famous for his role as *Tattoo*, in the television series *Fantasy Island* and the evil henchman *Nick Nack* in the *James Bond* movie *The Man with the Golden Gun*. To deal with bullying at school he would paint and he became the youngest

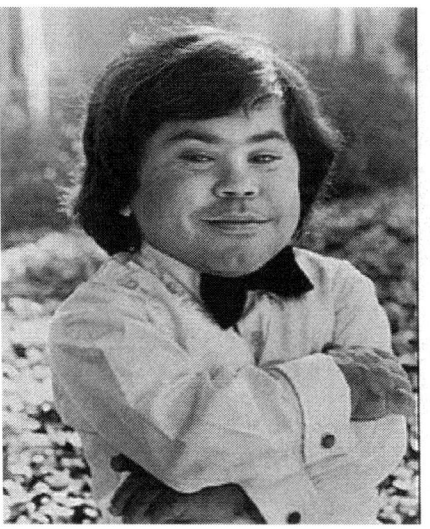

Hervé Villechaize, 1977

ever artist to have work displayed in the Museum of Paris. However, he suffered from chronic internal pains due to the condition and he sadly committed suicide aged 50 years old.

After setting a national record for the 100m, Gail Devers was picked for the 1988 Olympics. After a lot of expectation, she failed to make the finals, experiencing fatigue, muscle pulls, bouts of insomnia, fainting spells and migraines. Her hair then started to fall

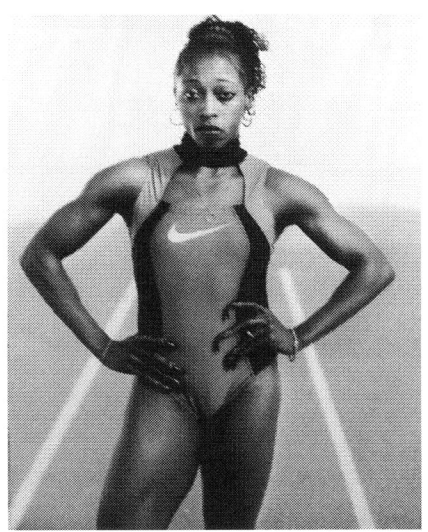

Gail Devers, 1996

out, her skin developed blotches and she suffered memory loss. Finally, after two years of illness, she was diagnosed with hyperthyroidism, also known as Graves' disease. This disorder describes the over-production of thyroid hormones. Thought to result from a combination of genetic and environmental factors, such as polymorphisms in HLA genes and particular infections and medications, these extra hormones lead to an imbalance in metabolism. Weight loss occurs, often accompanied by a ravenous appetite, fatigue, and a number of other symptoms. Treatment usually involves slowing down thyroid function or removing it and taking daily thyroid replacement hormone. However, Gail Dever's initial treatments caused more problems as large blisters appeared on her feet - at one point she was rushed to the hospital and doctors discussed amputating her feet. Following surgery to remove her thyroid, she returned to compete at the next two Olympics winning the 100m gold in both 1992 and 1996 and competing in the 2000 and 2004 games. There is a similar story with the Olympic skier Janica Kostelic. She suddenly collapsed with breathing problems whilst training on a glacier in Switzerland and had to be airlifted to a hospital. After being diagnosed with the same condition and having her thyroid removed at the beginning of 2005, she went on to win gold at the 2006 Winter Olympic Games in Turin – her fourth Olympic Gold – making her the then most successful female skier in the history of the Olympic Games.

The pair of adrenal glands (Lat. *ad*; above, *renes*; kidneys) are located just above the kidneys. These produce two steroids, aldosterone, which acts to conserve sodium ions and

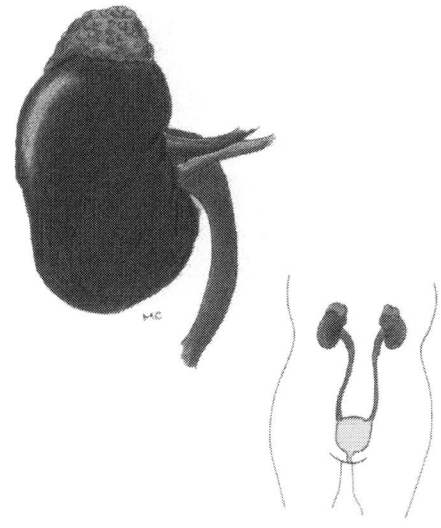

Adrenal gland

water in the body, and cortisol which increases blood glucose levels. They also secrete two hormones, epinephrine and norepinephrine, particularly during stress. When the adrenal glands become under-active Addison's disease occurs; when they are overactive Cushing's disease develops.

Addison's disease was first described in 1855 by the eminent British scientist, Thomas Addison at Guy's Hospital. Suffering from depression he sadly committed suicide. This disease may occur due to a genetic abnormality or may result from an autoimmune reaction, whereby the body's immune system attacks and destroys the adrenal tissue. A deficiency of aldosterone disrupts the kidney's ability to regulate water and salt balance leading to reduced blood pressure. In addition, the inability to produce corticosteroids can lead to an extreme sensitivity to insulin so that the level of sugar in the blood may fall dangerously low. A weakness of the muscles and the heart may also occur, and as a result the body may be unable to react properly under stress leading to possible severe medical complications. Significantly, the pituitary gland, in an attempt to stimulate the adrenal glands, becomes more active leading to increased melanin production and darkened "tanned" skin.

President John F. Kennedy was a well-cited sufferer of Addison's disease. A suspected occurrence of this same disease in his sister, Eunice Kennedy Shriver, implying a genetic link. At the age of 30, whilst in the UK, Kennedy was so ill that a doctor gave him

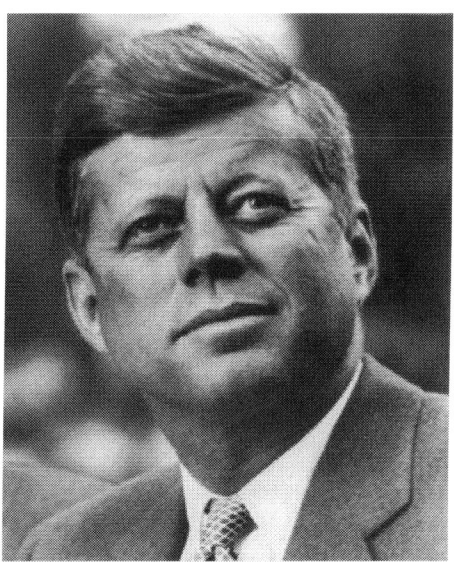

John F Kennedy, 1963

less than a year to live and he was even given the last rites by the ship's chaplain on his sea voyage home. However, 13 years later, when he ran for president, he appeared fit, healthy and "tanned". This no doubt influenced the voters, though his tanned appearance, rather than a sign of good health, may well have been a marker for his disease. Treatment usually involves lifelong cortisol to replace the steroids that the body no longer produces. Many photographs seem to show the typical swelling effects of the steroids, particularly in the face. Though the presidential staff at the time insisted he was a picture of health, the later release of his medical records show that he took steroids and a further cocktail of very strong pain medications, possibly to control the back pain resulting from osteoporosis that the steroids might have caused in the first place. Another person suggested by some to have suffered from Addison's disease was Jane Austen who died in 1817 at the age of 42. Her last words of "*Nothing, but death*", when asked by her sister Cassandra if there was anything she wanted, highlights the misery the disease could cause before the advent of modern-day steroid treatment. However, it is also possible that she may have succumbed to Hodgkin's disease, a form of lymphoma.

Cushing's syndrome, named after the American, Harvey Cushing, occurs when the adrenal glands become overactive, often due to a benign tumour, producing high levels of steroids, or else in response to cortisol medication. Cortisol controls the amount and distribution of body fat, and as a consequence, this disease typically leads to a large, round face and thickened trunk with arms and legs that are unusually slender in proportion. In addition, these steroids raise levels of testosterone which can lead to increased facial and body hair in women and balding in men. Elvis Presley was prescribed cortisone, amongst many other prescription drugs, to treat his back pain and he began to swell, especially in his face. Blood tests showed his adrenal glands were not working properly due to the high levels

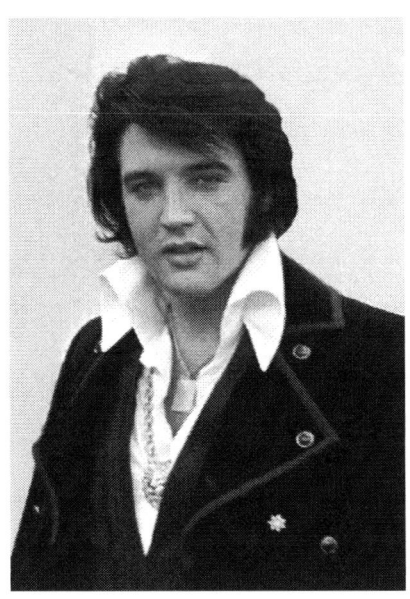

Elvis Presley, 1970

of this cortisone that may have further caused his gastric ulcer and liver damage. It has been suggested that Henry VIII may have suffered from Cushing's syndrome, simply on account of his rounded face and huge body shape seen in his portraits. The fact that this disorder can also cause irritability, depression, aggression, psychosis and impotence, might explain a few other things as well. However, a host of other possible disorders and conditions have also been suggested including the possibility of brain damage following a fall in a jousting contest or lead poisoning.

When rower Sir Steve Redgrave won his fifth Olympic gold medal at five consecutive games in Sydney 2000, he had a secret stash of sugar sachets sellotaped to the inside of his boat in case his blood sugar dropped too low. Just three years earlier he was diagnosed with type 2 diabetes. Disruptions in the insulin hormone, produced by the pancreas, lead to diabetes mellitus resulting in the body being unable to use glucose properly. This leads to increased levels of glucose sugar in the blood that can damage tissues. This excess glucose may also appear in the urine giving it a sweet smell, hence the name (Lat. *Mellitus*, sweet). People with type 2 diabetes either do not make enough insulin or cells in the body become more resistant to insulin leaving the body needing more and more insulin to try to keep blood sugar within a normal range. Though it can usually be managed through diet, exercise, and self-monitoring blood glucose, at least in the first few years following diagnosis, it is a progressive condition, and most people will eventually need

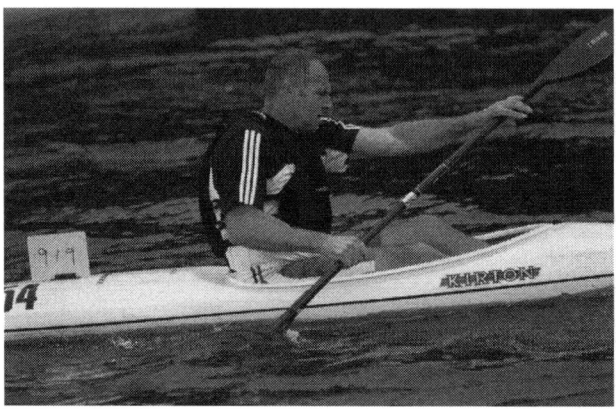

Sir Steven Redgrave in his first kayak race, 2011

to take insulin. Redgrave injects insulin around three times a week, down from 10 times a day when he was an athlete. A major worry of his is the increased risk of blindness as the peaks in sugar levels can damage sensitive cells such as those in the eyes. Sir Steven Redgrave certainly does not fit most people's preconceptions of someone with type 2 diabetes; the biggest risk factors are weight and lack of fitness - two of the things you would least associate with him. However, people of normal weight and fitness can still develop this disease as genes can also have an important role; studies show individuals with an affected parent have a 30 per cent chance of developing this disease.

Type 1 diabetes in most cases occurs from an autoimmune reaction where the body produces an immune response against insulin-producing cells in the pancreas and destroys them. Although not a classical Mendelian inherited disease, there is some genetic component. For example, a first-degree relative of an affected individual has about a 6 per cent chance of developing type 1 diabetes – higher than the 0.3 per cent in the general population. If untreated, very high blood glucose levels lead to dehydration, drowsiness, and serious illness which can be life-threatening. Fluctuations in blood sugar levels, even

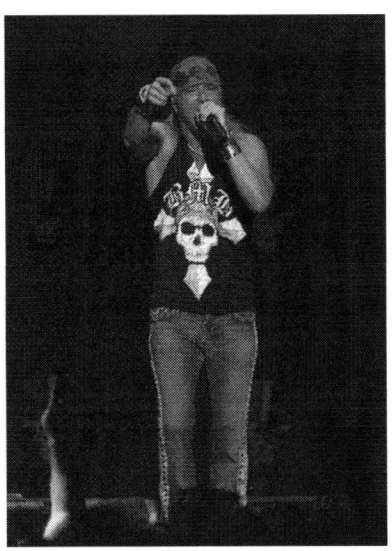

Bret Michaels, 2011

only mildly, over long periods of time can seriously affect the blood vessels leading to risks of angina, heart attacks, stroke and poor circulation as well as eye problems due to damage to the small arteries of the retina, kidney damage and nerve damage. This disease can occur at any age but is most commonly diagnosed from infancy to the late 30s. Bret Michaels, the lead vocalist of band *Poison*, was diagnosed with type I diabetes in early childhood and consequently takes four insulin injections and eight blood tests each day, according to his web site.

Former British Prime Minister, Theresa May was diagnosed much later in life with Type 1 diabetes in 2012, at the age of 56. This was after she had sought medical attention for sudden weight loss - a classic symptom of the condition along with increased thirst and tiredness. She has spoken about having to inject insulin up to five times a day and wears a monitoring patch that constantly checks the level of sugar in the blood. A fellow politician campaigning against her, Diane Abbott, revealed she suffered from type II diabetes that flared up badly during a 2017 election campaign, affecting her performances in some interviews. Returning to the Olympics, US swimmer Gary Hall Jr. was diagnosed with type 1 diabetes in 1999, having already won two Olympic gold medals in the 1996 Olympics. However, careful management of his condition allowed him to return to the following Olympics in Sydney 2000 winning two more gold medals. Competing as the oldest US male swimmer since 1924 at the following Athens 2004 games, he was able to defend his 50m freestyle title picking up another gold medal. He regularly speaks to young people with diabetes emphasising that their goals can be accomplished despite the fact that they live with the disease.

Metabolism of testosterone

The testes control maleness is by producing male sex steroid hormones known as androgens. These include testosterone and dihydrotestosterone that stimulate the development of the male sex organs in addition to other male characteristics. Mutations in the androgen receptor protein, that enables cells in the body to respond to these steroids, lead to androgen insensitivity syndrome. Mutations in the gene for enzymes important for producing either dihydrotestosterone and oestrogen cause 5-alpha-reductase deficiency, aromatase deficiency or congenital adrenal hyperplasia.

Mutations in the androgen receptor gene in a male person results in the individual's body being unable to react to testosterone. This leads to a hermaphrodite appearance, characterised by female characteristics but with testes that may be more or less evident. Referred to as androgen insensitivity syndrome, affecting around 1 in 13,000 individuals, the symptoms may be so subtle that they may go unnoticed until after puberty as most individuals do not menstruate and remain infertile. People with androgen insensitivity syndrome also tend to be taller, as the male Y chromosome can promote growth, and slimmer due to the effect of the small amounts of oestrogen produced by the testes that in

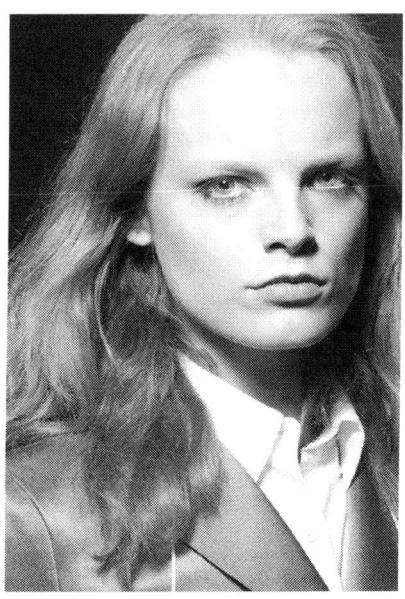

Hanne Gaby Odiele

addition can stimulate breast growth and a curvaceous figure. Also, due to low levels of androgens, girls with this disorder will generally not suffer from acne and often present with clear skin, luxuriantly thick scalp hair and little body hair. Many women with this disorder may be drawn to occupations such as modelling or acting. The well-known model for many of the top fashion powerhouses, Hanne Gaby Odiele, was 2 weeks old when doctors, after running a routine blood test, told her parents she was genetically male. Further tests revealed she had internal testes instead of a uterus and ovaries. Though having spent large parts of her childhood in and out of hospitals undergoing treatments and operations, it was not until 17 years of age that Hanna herself actually discovered she had condition; her parents and doctors had tried to keep secret from her. *Doctors think they have to 'normalize' the baby,'* says Odiele, who is dedicated to stopping non-consensual genital surgeries on intersex children. In 2016, The United Nations urged that these practices should be classified as torture.

A number of well-known women in history may have suffered from androgen insensitivity syndrome. The gender of Joan of Arc raised speculation during her life. An

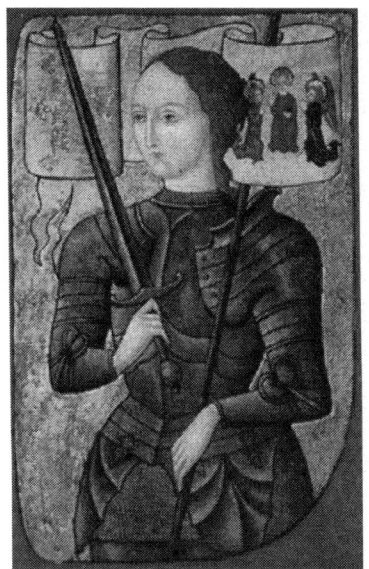

Joan of Arc

206

investigation following her execution in 1431, which received testimonies from over 100 witnesses, established that she had well developed breasts, no pubic hair, and had never menstruated.

Born in 1838 in Saint-Jean-d'Angély, France, Herculine Barbin was raised as a girl and attended a convent school for girls. As she moved into adolescence, however, her breasts failed to develop, facial hair started to appear, and she suffered painful abdominal pains. Aged 18 she became a school-mistress and began a relationship with the headmistress' daughter, Sara. One day, a doctor was called to check her abdominal pains and informed her that she had descending testes. He abruptly reassigned her sex as male, suggesting the new name of Abel.

It would appear that Herculine had been born with 5-alpha-reductase deficiency. 5-alpha-reductase is an enzyme important in converting testosterone to the more potent androgen, dihydrotestosterone. This is responsible for early male sex characteristics, while testosterone influences masculinisation during adolescence. A lack of 5-alpha-reductase and dihydrotestosterone in male embryos leads to a failure of genital growth and development of female characteristics until adolescence when testosterone takes over and masculinisation occurs with testes descending and the growth of facial hair. Cast out from her job and losing her relationship with Sara, Herculine went to Paris to find work in various menial jobs. Sadly, she committed suicide a few years later leaving a book of memoirs which has since formed the basis for the novel *Middlesex* by Jeffrey Eugenides. Herculine Barbin's birthday, the 8th November, is now internationally designated as the Intersex Solidarity Day. This condition is particularly common in certain remote parts of the Dominican Republic; colloquially known as "testes-at-twelve", as many as 1 per cent of children regarded as female have their gender reassigned at puberty. Inherited autosomal recessively, all these individuals can trace their ancestry to a single woman, by the name of Altagracia Carrasco, who carried the mutation and lived in the mid-nineteenth century.

Another enzyme, aromatase, is responsible for turning testosterone into oestrogen. Mutations in the gene for this enzyme leads to individuals producing increased levels of testosterone and reduced levels of oestrogen. Females born with aromatase deficiency can show ambiguous genitalia at birth but typically have normal internal reproductive organs. In adolescence, females often fail to develop secondary sexual characteristics, such as breast growth and may develop acne and excessive body and facial hair. They may also be taller due to the effect of testosterone on bone growth. There are cases where the high levels of testosterone produced by a foetus with this disorder, has passed across the placenta to the mother who consequently develops facial and body hair, acne, and a deep voice during pregnancy, all of which disappear soon after delivery.

Aristotle first noted more than 2,000 years ago, that the female spotted hyenas are bigger and more aggressive than the males. This is due to the species containing a mutant aromatase gene, further leading to the females having an enlarged clitoris which also serves as a birth canal; a number of hyenas die during birth. Packs of spotted hyenas are led by a

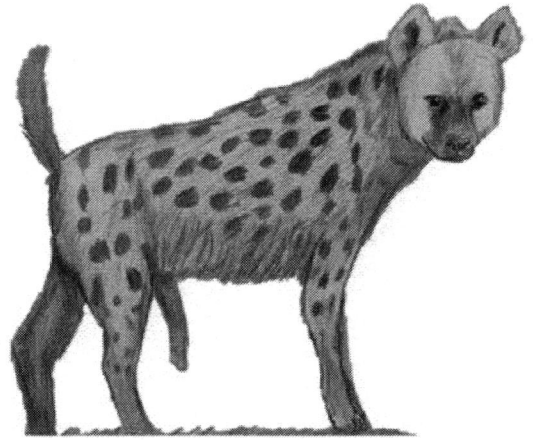

Female spotted hyena

single alpha female, whilst the highest-ranked male in the group is still subordinate to the lowest-ranked female. This is illustrated in the *Disney* movie *The Lion King*. The script-writers and artists spent some time observing the animals before creating *Shenzi* the female spotted hyena, who is the biggest and strongest, and leader of the pack.

Congenital adrenal hyperplasia, results from a lack of the enzyme, 21-hydroxylase, needed by the adrenal gland to make the hormones cortisol and aldosterone. Without these hormones, the body produces more androgen causing male characteristics to appear early in males or inappropriately in females. Autosomal recessively inherited, boys with this disorder enter puberty early, sometimes at 2-3 years of age, developing a deep voice and pubic hair. Females inheriting such a mutation, however, can also develop male characteristics such as a deep voice and excessive body and facial hair. However, they tend to have normal female reproductive organs through their genitals may look both male and female. Lisa Lee Dark, the Welsh opera singer, was raised as a boy until 19 years of age when she finally realised that she had been born with the condition and was biologically female. In 2008, Christiane Völling, a nurse in Düsseldorf, became the first person to successfully sue for non-consensual sex-reassignment. Born in 1959 with indeterminate external genitalia due to this condition, Völling was raised as a boy. However, at the age of 18, when in hospital to have her appendix removed, doctors found her to have a uterus, fallopian tubes and ovaries but no testis. Without her being properly informed, these were all completely removed the following year leaving her with no sex organs. Though Völling continued to live as a man for a time, she later transitioned to live as a woman. It was not until 2006, that she finally realised she was intersex and discovered in her medical records she'd had a previously concealed female XX chromosomal diagnosis, and that the nature of her earlier surgery had made it impossible for her to live as a woman.

# METABOLIC DISORDERS

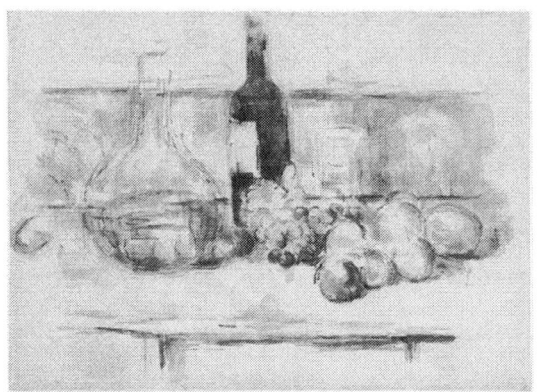

*What is food to one man may be fierce poison to others.*

Lucretius (99 BC – 55 BC)

Metabolism is the set of chemical transformations that occur within us. Most of these chemical reactions require a catalyst to get started – a function performed by enzymes. These are protein molecules, produced by our genes, that drive chemical reactions within our bodies and cells without changing themselves.

There are many different diseases in which individuals lack a particular enzyme involved in converting various substances into other products, i.e. metabolism. Termed 'inborn errors of metabolism' by the British physician, Sir Archibald Garrod, in the early 1900s, the diseases highlight the fact that one gene produces one enzyme protein. In other words, a mutation in one particular gene will only affect the one particular protein produced by that gene. While seemingly obvious now, this was a very astute observation at the time and helped pave the way for understanding the basis of genes and inheritance.

Metabolic diseases result from the loss of any one of a number of enzymes required for efficient metabolism of various substances. An inability to properly metabolise some carbohydrates can lead to lactose intolerance, glycogen storage diseases or galactosemia, while inherited defects in the metabolism of specific amino acids can lead to disorders such as phenylketonuria and maple syrup urine disease. Mutations in genes disrupting the ability to metabolise specific fats and lipids result in disorders such as Tay-Sachs disease while disorders resulting from an inability to break down some of the products of DNA include Lesch-Nyhan syndrome and gout. All of these diseases can either lead to the accumulation of toxic substances in the body or else a deficiency in the specific biological compounds this enzyme is important in producing.

Mammals have evolved a clever way to shorten the length of time an offspring is dependent on the mother. This involves a mechanism in which the gene for lactase, needed for the metabolism of the lactose sugar found in milk, is turned off at the end of the weaning period. So, while young mammals are able to digest milk from the mother, they will reach a stage shortly after weaning when the consumption of milk will cause cramps and diarrhoea.

This also occurs in humans where a child's bodily production of the lactase enzyme decreases dramatically after the first couple of years of life, resulting in lactose intolerance. Almost two-thirds of the global population are lactose intolerant. Most of the population of Europe and the US would still be milk intolerant if it were not for one or more individuals living in present day Hungary 7,500 years ago. Being born with a mutation bypassing the normal shutdown in lactase production enabled these individuals to consume milk throughout their adult lives. This would have been a considerable evolutionary advantage, following the first domestication of animals, as milk became a valuable source of nutrition. While most of Western Europeans have inherited this mutation and can safely consume milk, many in African and Asian countries have remained lactose intolerant.

In the 1930s, the Norwegian physician, Ivar Asbjørn Følling, noticed a disease in children living near his hometown of Oslo. Seemingly healthily growing infants would, at some point, stop developing normally and drift into irreversible mental retardation. Another thing he noticed was that these affected infants produced urine with a characteristic musty odour now known to be associated with the disease. He, therefore,

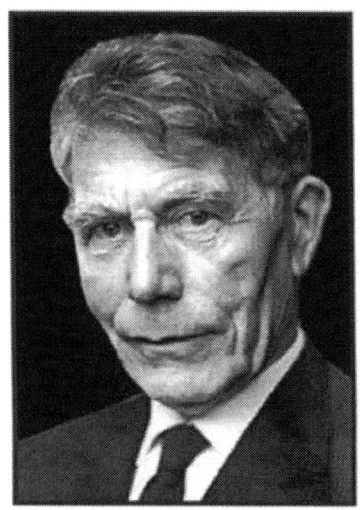

Ivar Asbjørn Følling

speculated whether this might be reflective of a defect in metabolism and so set about seeing if the musty smell might derive from any unbroken down products in the urine of the children. He found that the urine of all affected children contained phenylketone. This is a derivative of the amino acid phenylalanine, suggesting a defect in the metabolism of this amino acid. Følling's pioneering work served two life-saving purposes: it allowed the diagnosis of this disorder, and also provided the cure, which simply involved restricting the diets of those affected children to only those foods containing low levels of phenylalanine. Now termed phenylketonuria - referring to phenyketones in the urine - the disorder results from inherited mutations in the gene which produces the enzyme needed to convert the amino acid phenylalanine into the amino acid tyrosine. The resulting higher levels of phenylalanine in the blood harm brain development and can lead to mental retardation if not treated. In addition, some of the excess phenylalanine is converted into a phenylketone called phenylpyruvic acid, which, when excreted in the sweat and the urine, gives the characteristic musty odour. Many consider Følling to be among the most important medical scientists to have not received a Nobel Prize.

Perhaps one of the first reports of phenylketonuria was by the Nobel prize-winning American author, Pearl Sydenstricker Buck, in her book *The Child Who Never Grew*. Here she described how her 3-year-old daughter in the 1920s started to become severely mentally retarded in early childhood. She wrote: "*Although the child was beautiful, her mind was not developing. I remember when she was only 3 months old, she lay in her basket on the sun deck of a ship. I had taken her there for the morning air. The people who promenaded on deck often stopped to look at her, and my pride grew as they spoke of her unusual beauty and of the intelligent look of her deep, blue eyes. I do not know at what moment the growth of her intelligence stopped.*" Years after Ivar Asbjørn Følling's discovery she reported that she remembered the characteristic smell.

Tay-Sachs disease occurs due to mutations disrupting the function of an enzyme needed to break down specific fats known as lipids which then accumulate in tissues, particularly neurons that use this type of lipid. Children with this disease become progressively retarded and develop spasticity, paralysis, dementia, and blindness, ending with early death, usually by 4 years of age. Autosomal recessive inherited, this disease is most common in families of Eastern European Jewish origin, where as many as 1 in 45 are carriers of the mutant gene compared to the general incidence of 1 in 300. This disease has been described in the Ashkenazi Jewish population as early as the 15th century; the continuing high incidence suggests a possible heterozygous advantage in this population. There is some evidence that carriers of the Tay-Sachs disease gene have an increased resistance to Tuberculosis, and one idea is that Jewish populations in the past were often confined to urban areas high in *Mycobacterium tuberculosis* bacteria, and were consequently placed under selective pressures to evolve resistance to the disease.

This high prevalence of Tay-Sachs disease, and other genetic disorders, in some Jewish communities, has led to the establishment of the Committee for Prevention of Genetic Diseases to develop routine genetic testing of young Jewish people worldwide. This was started in the 1980s by Rabbi Joseph Ekstein, who lost four of his five children to the disease. People tested are given a telephone number and a PIN, but are not told their results. Then, when a shidduch - an introduction of marriageable singles - is suggested, the candidates can phone the organisation, enter both their PINs and find out whether their union could result in severely disabled children. Although sometimes receiving criticism, such practices have led to a sharp decline in the occurrence of Tay-Sachs disease in Jewish communities. In New York, it was reported that the incidence of Tay-Sachs in the 1970s had fallen by more than 90 per cent among this community due in a large part to this initiative.

Purines and pyrimidines are the bases found in the nucleotides making up DNA and RNA; Adenine and Guanine are purines whereas Thymine and Cytosine are pyrimidines. These are broken down in different pathways; pyrimidines into beta-amino acids and ammonia, while purines are degraded into urate which is further processed and excreted as uric acid. Lesch-Nyhan syndrome results from inheriting a mutation in a gene involved in purine metabolism leading to increased levels of uric acid. This results in arthritis and severe neurological problems including mental retardation, and self-mutilating behaviour involving biting of the lips, tongue and fingers. This disease was first described in 1964 by Dr Michael Lesch, a medical student, and Dr William Nyhan, a paediatrician, at Johns Hopkins Hospital, Baltimore, when they identified symptoms in two affected brothers aged four and eight.

Gout can also result from high concentrations of urate in the blood leading to uric acid crystals forming inside joints, often in the big toe, producing intense pain. The word gout possibly derives from the Greek "*podagra*" (*pod*; foot, *agra*; trap). Although most cases appear to be the product of diet, mutations in certain genes involved in the metabolism of the purine component of DNA may lead to an inherited predisposition to gout. For example, one such gene coding for an enzyme degrading uric acid, when mutated, can lead to an increased predisposition for gout and renal failure. This may explain why certain populations, such as people of the Pacific Islands, and the Maoris of New Zealand, show higher occurrence of this ailment. Incidences of gout in 3,000- year-old skeletons on some Pacific islands are suggestive of a founder effect with the genes responsible for this condition possibly having been carried to the islands by the early settlers.

One possible example of familial gout was in Charles V of Spain (a Habsburg, hence the jaw), one of the most powerful rulers of all time during his reign from 1516-1556. His gout first became evident aged 28 and as he grew older the attacks increased in frequency and severity. Towards the end of his life, he had to be carried around in a specially designed chair as he was barely able to walk or use his hands. Recent analyses of his mummified body revealed high levels of urate deposits confirming his gout. Charles passed on his vast empire, and his ailment, to his son Phillip. Also suffering severely, Phillip supposedly rarely complained about his condition which he regarded as punishment from God for "*not being diligent enough to eradicate the protestant heresy*".

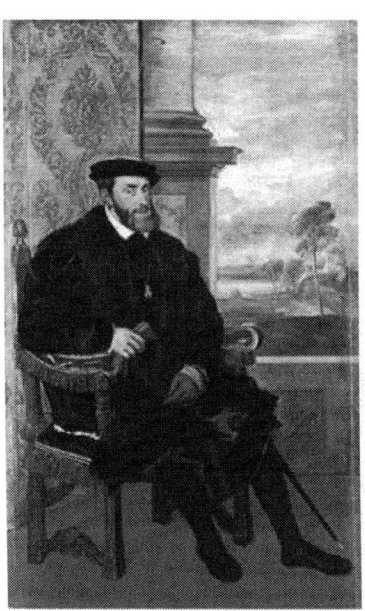

Charles V of Spain by Lambert Sustris, 1548

# VISUAL DISORDERS

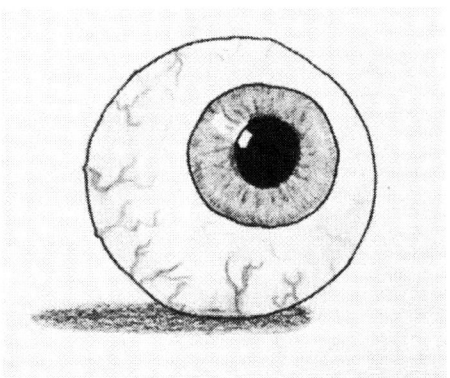

Painting is a blind man's profession. He never paints what he sees, but what he feels

Pablo Picasso

Eye colour is determined by the amount of melanin in the iris of the eye; people with brown eyes have more melanin, which absorbs more light and causes the iris to look brown while less melanin causes more blue light reflects out. Brown is the most widespread eye colour in the world. One study has suggested that all humans had brown eyes until one individual living some 6,000 to 10,000 years ago, acquired a specific genetic mutation that turned off the ability to produce high levels of melanin in the iris. Blue eye colour is more confined to Northern and Eastern Europe while Green, one of the rarest eye colours, is fairly common among Pashtuns, as seen in Sharbat Gula the *Afghan Girl* from the June 1985 cover of

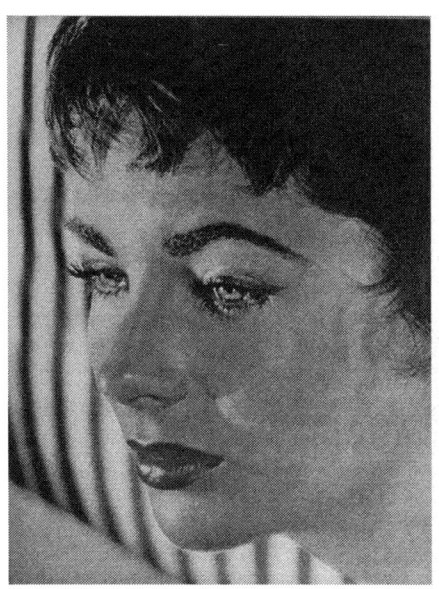

Elizabeth Taylor, 1954

*National Geographic*), as well as people of Celtic, Germanic and Slavic descent. The British film star Elizabeth Taylor had rare violet coloured eyes. This is thought to be due to a genetic mutation in a particular gene, which causes a specific amount of melanin producing a striking eye colour and may additionally cause double eye lashes as well as heart problems in some individuals.

Previous assumptions were that the inheritance of eye colour was relatively simple involving only one gene with a version (allele) for brown eyes dominant over blue eyes. However, the genetic basis for eye colour is actually far more complex and is a polygenetic trait, controlled by at least 16 different genes interacting with each other to give the various colour shades. As such, almost any parent-child combination of eye colours can occur.

Some individuals have different coloured eyes, known as heterochromia (Gr, *hetero*, different; *chromo*, colours). A number of movie actors have eye colour irregularities, the presence of which can create a more striking appearance. For example, Dan Aykroyd, Demi More and Jane Seymour have one green eye and one brown or hazel eye. This is often genetic in origin, and often autosomal dominant inherited. The actress Kate Bosworth has a section of hazel colour in only part of her right otherwise blue eye. This is known as sectoral heterochromia where individuals show different colours within a single eye. While some casting agents insisted that she wore coloured contact lenses to cover it, for *Superman Returns* she was allowed to go "natural"; as a result, *Barbie* manufactured an accompanying *Louis Lane* Doll with the same pigment defect. Simon Pegg and Elizabeth

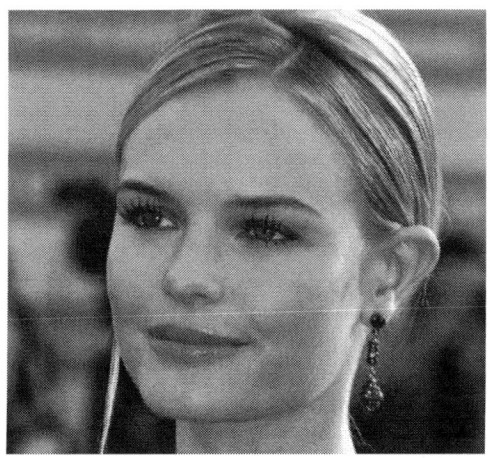

Kate Bosworth

Berkley also have similar brown patches in their right eyes, while Jessica Cauffiel and Henry Cavill have patches of brown pigmentation in their left eyes. Christopher Walken and Benedict Cumberbatch have eyes that are both a mixture of blue and green. There are dozens more actors and actresses with similar eye pigment disorders. Heterochromia is also particularly common in some breeds of dogs such as Dalmatians and Border Collies.

David Bowie, however, did not have heterochromia and explained that his discoloured eye was the result of a permanently dilated pupil following a punch he received in a fight over a girl when he was at school. The differently coloured eyes of Mila Kulis are the result of an early inflammation of her iris that led to a cataract that gave the eye a different appearance; this has since been corrected. Marilyn Manson does not have heterochromia or any iris injuries but uses differently coloured contact lenses to give this appearance.

A developmental defect of the iris can result in a pupil that is misshapen, often resembling a keyhole. Known as a coloboma (Gr. *koloboma*; defect), it may or may not affect vision and is caused by changes in different genes involved in the early development of the eye. Similarly, to heterochromia, there are several actors and actresses with this. For example, the Polish-American actress and model, Karolina Wydra, was born with this

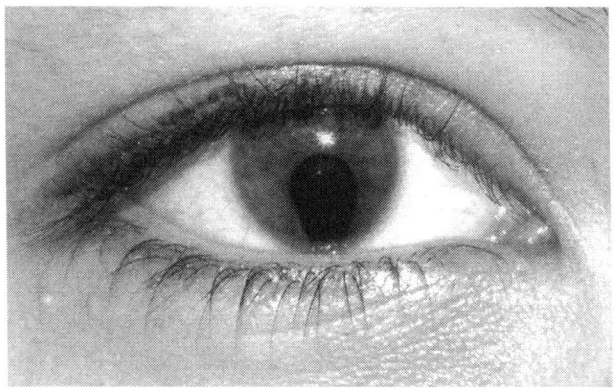

Colobma

defect in her left eye. She played *Dominika Petrova* on the *Fox* medical drama series *House* and the vampire *Violet Mazurski* on the fantasy series *True Blood*.

Light entering the eye is focused by the lens onto a light-sensitive panel of cells known as the retina at the rear of the eye. It is here that the light is detected and converted into electrical signals by photoreceptor cells of which there are two types: cone cells are responsible for sharp vision and colour vision while rod cells, named for their cylindrical shape, are highly sensitive to light and so are responsible for night and peripheral vision. These cells transmit the light signals to the brain via the optic nerve.

Defects in cone cells result in colour blindness and day blindness describing an extreme sensitivity to light. One inherited disease characterised by this is Stargardt's disease. Here mutations in a gene, producing a protein involved in providing energy to retinal cells, leads to the gradual deterioration of cone cells and central vision, along with the ability to perceive colours while leaving peripheral vision intact. Inherited autosomal recessively and affecting around 1 in 10,000 people, problems with sight begin in childhood with light sensitivity, wavy vision, blind spots, blurriness, impaired colour vision, and difficulty adjusting when moving from light to dark environments.

The athlete Marla Runyan, though having competed in the Olympic final in Sydney 2000 for the 1,500 meters run, suffers from Stargardt's disease. Her vision was perfectly normal until she was about 9 years old, at which time she began to experience problems seeing the blackboard in school and reading books. As a result of this condition Marla Runyan is legally blind but is still able to see shadows and peripheral details. In her biography, *No Finish Line*, she recalls being amazed to discover that other hurdlers could see all ten hurdles on the track when she could barely see the first one! It was this that led her to switch to distance running. In the 2010 Winter Olympics, the Canadian cross-country skier Brian McKeever, who also suffers from this disease, became the first winter athlete to compete in both the Paralympic and Olympic games.

A loss of rod cells in the retina or disruption in their ability to respond to light can lead to night-blindness, where individuals find it difficult or impossible to see in relatively low light. Retinitis pigmentosa, one of the most common forms of inherited retinal degeneration affecting around 1 in 3,000 individuals, is typically characterised by the progressive loss of rod cells. This leads to night-blindness followed later by a reduction of the peripheral visual field, known as tunnel vision. Over 40 different genes are known to cause this disease when mutated and consequently, the disease shows many different patterns of inheritance depending upon which gene is affected. Former child actor Isaac Lidsky who played the role of *Weasel* in *Saved by the Bell* was diagnosed with this at age 13. Gradually, over the next 10 years, he became completely blind. Two of his sisters also inherited the same gene and condition. Giving up acting, he completed a degree in Applied Mathematics and Computer Science at Harvard followed by a degree in Law at Harvard - in 2008 he became the first legally blind US Supreme Court clerk. An author, motivational speaker and highly successful entrepreneur, he is also the Chairman and President of the *Hope for Vision* foundation.

Liverpool comedian and actor Chris McCausland, who was also born with this hereditary eye disease, explained how it felt like a gradual loss of his sight all the way through his childhood. He said that he could not read the letters on the blackboard at school and his vision became progressively blurred until eventual complete blindness as a teenager. It was only after being forced to give up his job as a website designer in his 20s that he turned to stand-up comedy. In 2020, he appeared on an episode of *8 Out of 10 Cats Does Countdown* together with sighted panellists competing to solve maths problems and anagrams, simply using his memory.

Uncontrolled growth of the retina, leading to a cancer of this tissue, can result from inherited mutations in a gene coding for a protein that normally functions in cells as a tumour suppressor, acting as a brake on cell division. This causes a disease, known as retinoblastoma, that can affect either one or both eyes, and usually occurs in childhood.

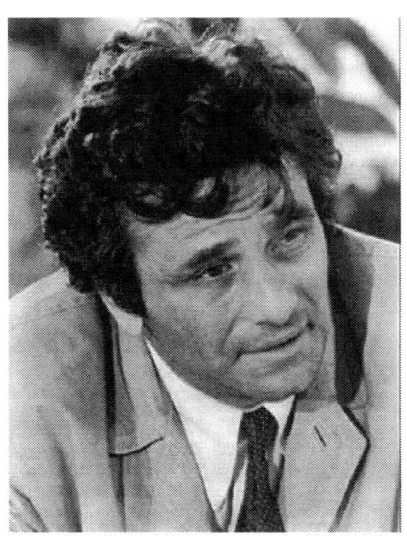

Peter Falk, 1973

Peter Falk, the American actor, best known for his role as *Lieutenant Columbo*, suffered from retinoblastoma as a child, lost his right eye at the age of 3 and subsequently wore a glass eye. The late English comedienne, actress and writer Caroline Ahern was also partially sighted in one eye as a result of suffering this in childhood, as well as her brother who inherited the same gene.

Short-sightedness, known as Myopia, is the most common eye problem in the world. Affecting a quarter of the population, it occurs when the lens of the eye is unable to flatten properly causing light entering the eye to focus in front of the retina. This leaves the individual with trouble seeing things that are far away. This visual defect usually presents during the pre-teen years, worsens gradually as the eye grows during adolescence, and then levels off as a person reaches adulthood. The risk of developing this condition is greater for children of affected parents, though the condition does not have a clear pattern of inheritance. Myopia is, therefore, a complex condition involving hundreds of genes. Interestingly, this is very common in some East Asian countries, where the condition affects up to 90 per cent of young adults. It has been suggested that the artistic style of Impressionism may owe its existence to the poor eyesight associated with myopia. Artists such as Monet, Renoir and Degas supposedly suffered from short-sightedness to varying degrees which may have influenced their painting style. It has been claimed that some impressionist artists removed their spectacles while painting in order to achieve the desired effect.

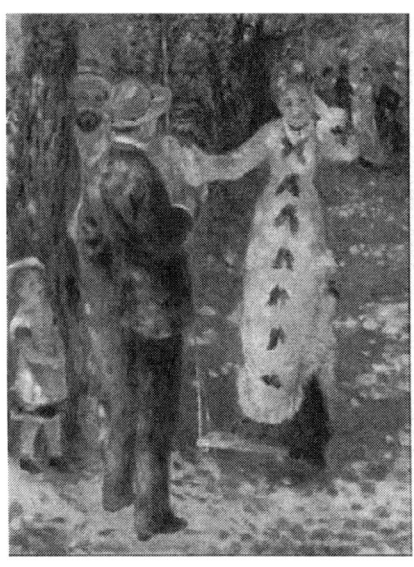

*The swing* by Pierre-Auguste Renoir, 1876

John Milton, considered one of the greatest poets of the English language, wrote his epic poem *Paradise Lost* (1667) after he became blind. It was while he was in his 30s, that he felt his sight getting weak and dull until by the age of 43 he was totally blind. He suffered from glaucoma (Gr. *glaukos*; blue-grey – possibly first used to describe cataracts), a term used for a group of diseases that can lead to damage of the eye's optic nerve resulting in blindness. This disease generally occurs when fluid pressure inside the eye becomes too high, causing damage to the optic nerve. Affecting around 1 in 200 people it does not show a simple Mendelian inheritance though relatives of people who have the condition do have a higher risk of developing the condition themselves. As such, relatives are usually advised to have their eye pressures tested at regular intervals, with the NHS providing free eye

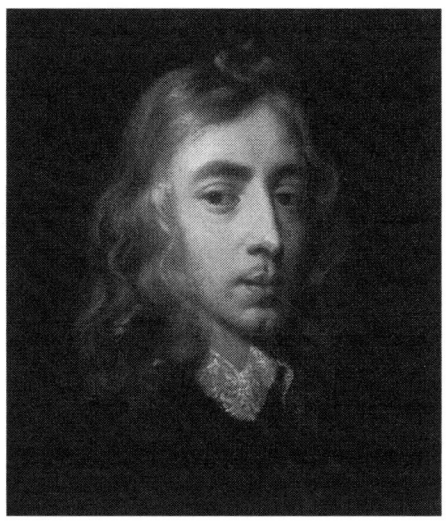

John Milton, (1608-1674)

checks for people with an affected parent. There are a small number of cases of familial glaucoma where mutations in several specific genes lead to a higher risk, usually at an earlier age. The most common mutation is found in a gene which produces a protein involved in pressure regulation in the eye.

Glaucoma can be acute, where sight is lost suddenly, or it can develop slowly, sometimes over decades. The latter, sometimes referred to as 'the silent sight thief', leads to a gradual, often unnoticed, impairment of vision taking place over a long period of time. Similarly, to John Milton, the great Argentinian writer Jorge Luis Borges lost his sight to glaucoma, which he may have inherited from his father who had become blind in middle age, as had other relations on his father's side of the family. *"In my case, that slow nightfall, that slow loss of sight, began when I began to see. It has continued since 1899 without dramatic moments, a slow nightfall that has lasted more than three-quarters of a century"*. In contrast, Johann Sebastian Bach went blind suddenly, aged 65, apparently with a blinding flash. He died months after an unsuccessful operation on his eyes in 1750. He probably suffered from an acute form of the blindness, known as acute (closed-angle) glaucoma that results from a sudden increase

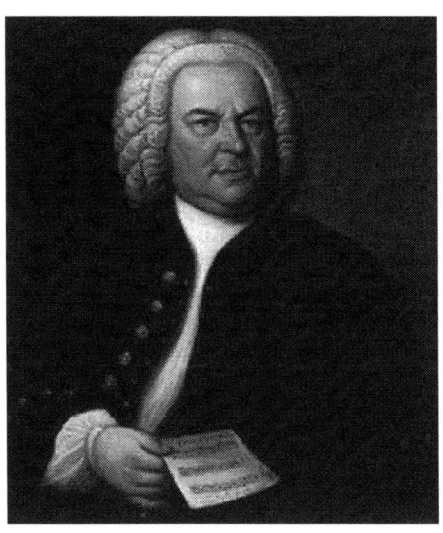

Johann Sebastian Bach by Elias Gottlob Haussmann, 1746

in eye pressure. Symptoms can last for a few hours accompanied with severe eye pain, leading to either permeant damage in some, while others recover and may then suffer multiple subsequent attacks. One of the typical symptoms is seeing bright circles or rings around a light source, referred to as 'halos' that are especially noticeable at night-time. It has been suggested that such 'halos', evident in some paintings of van Gogh's such as the *'The Night Café'* or *'The Starry Night'* could indicate acute glaucoma. However, hypotheses surrounding the mental and visual health of van Gogh are many and varied.

People with a colour vision deficiency find it difficult to identify and distinguish between certain colours. This is sometimes referred to as 'colour blindness', though this is not total colour blindness. The most common deficiency is red-green colour blindness. This generally affects males as the genes for two of the photoreceptors involved in this disorder are on the X chromosome; around 8 per cent of males and 0.4 per cent of females in the UK are affected. This results in a variable degree of reduced perception of red, orange, green and blue. Many people are unaware of their colour deficiencies, which are often only revealed by tests such as an Ishihara diagram in which an individual is asked to identify numbers contained within images made up of different coloured dots. Many people with a colour vision deficiency have few, if any, difficulties and can do most normal activities including driving. However, certain jobs, such as pilots, train drivers, electricians and air traffic controllers, may require accurate colour-recognition. In 2009, four of the 32 snooker competitors who took part in the World Snooker Championship at The Crucible suffered from various degrees of colour blindness: Mark Williams, three times world champion, Peter Ebdon, once world champion, Mark Allen and Stephen Lee. All, have on occasion,

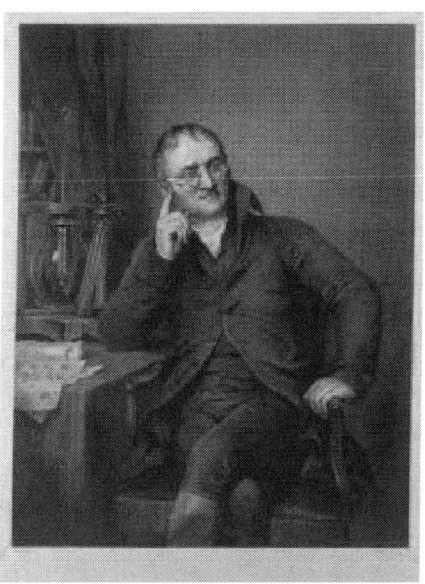

John Dalton. Line engraving by W H Worthington, 1823

had to clarify with a referee the colour of a particular ball.

John Dalton, one of England's most renowned chemists, was red-green colour blind and was one of the first to describe the condition. He correctly surmised that it must be hereditary since his brother had the same visual defect. However, he was mistakenly convinced that this defect resulted from the lens of his eye being tinted blue and he requested that after his death in 1844 his eyes be removed and examined to confirm this. Though his lenses were found not to be tinted, for many years colour blindness was called 'Daltonism', after him. However, the potential problems associated with red-green colour blindness were not widely appreciated until 1875, when a train accident in Sweden was attributed to the driver's colour blindness.

Interestingly, while as many as 8 percent of North Europeans are affected by this disorder, it is far less common in other ethnic groups, especially those closer to the equator. One possible reason is that colour blind people may have better night vision and this may

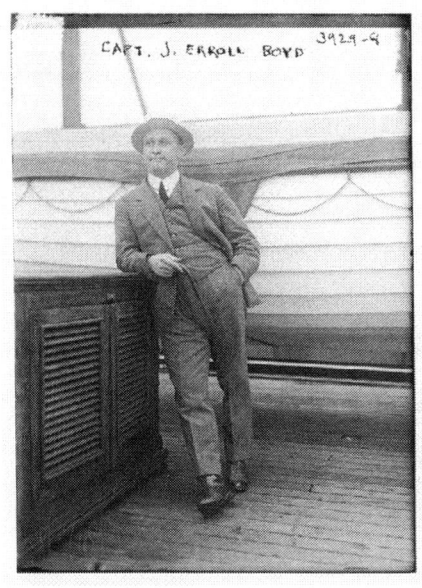

James Erroll Dunsford Boyd, 1916

have been an evolutionary advantage for people living closer to the poles in areas with longer twilight periods. For example, one can imagine this might have improved hunting skills such areas. The famous Canadian World War I combat pilot and aviation daredevil, James Erroll Boyd, was turned down by the Royal Flying Corps because of his colour blindness. However, he was accepted by the Royal Naval Air Service, where he excelled at flying night missions. He also became the first person to fly across the North Atlantic, in 1930, outside the summer season. He later recalled: *"Boy, it was dark! I felt as though I was piloting a car in a coal mine."*

There are numerous artists who were supposedly colour-blind leading to their individual styles. Interestingly, many of them are still renowned for their use of colours. Ferdinand Léger, whose paintings were characterised by bold often drab colours in geometric forms, would have to ask his wife for the names of some colours when preparing his palette. Often thought of as the founder of Modern Art for developing the use of colours, Piet Mondrian, is also thought to have had this; using only three fundamental colours of red, yellow and blue - but never green. Other landscape artists such as John Constable, from examinations of their colouring, have also been suggested to have had a degree of colour-blindness. One test is to look for something in a painting that is typically red, such as red roof tiles and see to what degree the painter has used green. These differences in colour perception may have also influenced comic book art with a number of artists known to have the visual defect. Albert Uderzo, co-creator and illustrator of *Asterix* series, for example, was found he had red-green colour blindness around the age of 12 and would use labels on his colours .

Total colour blindness is known as achromatopsia, where individuals are only able to differentiate shades of grey. This can result from an inherited inability of cone cells to transmit signals and react to light. Many of the inhabitants of the small coral island of Pingelap, in the Western Pacific Ocean, are unable to distinguish any colours. A freak storm in the eighteenth century killed most of the islanders leaving only around twenty women and a handful of men including a young chief who happened to be a carrier of the gene for achromatopsia. Consequently, around a third of the atoll's 3,000 inhabitants now carry the gene leading to 6 per cent of the population suffering from the disorder. There are

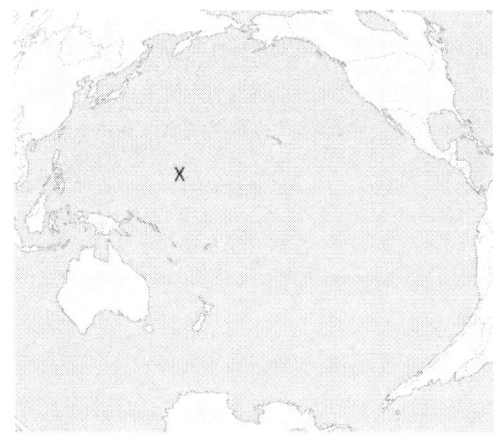

Pingelap

some suggestions that individuals with the disorder are more successful at night fishing.

When Canada became a royal province in 1663, there was an unfavourable ratio of six male colonists to every female. With a view to reducing this imbalance and to ensuring the stability of the colony, the French King Louis XIV devised a program whereby over 700 young single French women were sent out between 1663 and 1673. Most of these women were orphans who had already been placed under the care of the king and so became known as the '*Filles du Roy*', or '*King's daughters*'. Many of the 5 million French-Canadians living in Quebec province are descendants of these women. One, however, carried a single nucleotide change in her mitochondrial DNA coding for a disease called

Leber's hereditary optic neuropathy. This leads to permanent damage of the optic nerve and irreversible blindness in young adulthood. Marrying one of the colonists in Quebec City in 1669, she had five daughters who also all married in or near Quebec City. As this is a mitochondrial inherited disease it is passed exclusively through the mothers and today, as many as 90 per cent of French-Canadians affected with Leber's hereditary optic

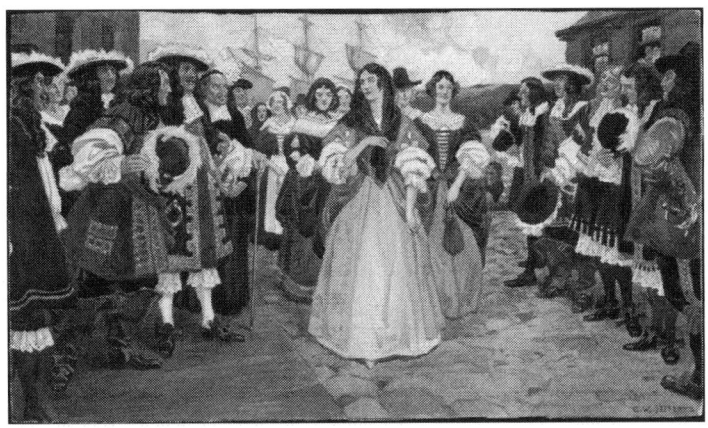

The arrival of the French girls at Quebec, 1667. By Charles William Jefferys

neuropathy can trace their ancestry back to this one woman. This is another example of a founder effect.

The renowned German ophthalmologist Theodor Karl Gustav von Leber was also the first to describe another form of blindness two years earlier in 1869, since known as Leber's congenital amaurosis (Gr. *Amauroun*, darken, referring to blindness without visible change in the eye). This is an inherited defect in both rod and cone cells resulting in blindness from birth. There are almost 20 different causal genes leading to the abnormal development of both types of photoreceptor cells. Scott MacIntyre, the American singer, songwriter, and pianist, has only 2 per cent vision as a result of this form of blindness. Another singer born with this disorder is Singaporean, Kelvin Tan Wei Lian, who was a

231

street busker before winning a national competition and securing a recording contract.

Albinism, resulting from defects in melanin production also leads to visual defects,

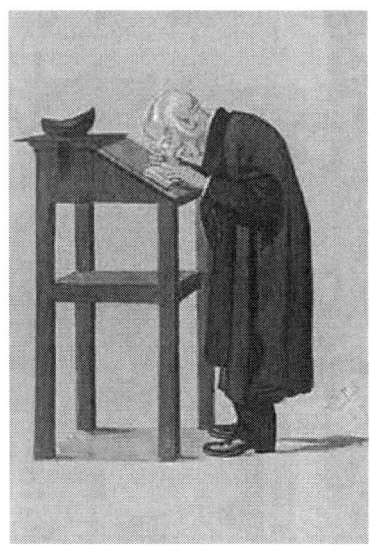

Dr William Spooner by Leslie Ward 1898

with individuals generally showing sensitivity to light due to the lack of any melanin in the iris important for reducing the intensity of light entering the eye. However, the major vision defects in people with albinism result from an abnormality in an area of the retina important for sharp vision such as reading. This tissue requires melanin for the proper development of nerve connections between the retina and the brain. When these connections are disrupted involuntary movements of the eyes, known as nystagmus, can occur in addition to strabismus where the eyes are unable to align together, sometimes referred to as 'cross-eyed'. Dr Spooner, the famous Oxford classicist, may have had this condition as a result of his albinism. His nystagmus may have caused a jumbling of information from the printed page which led to his famous speech aberration, now referred to as spoonerism.

Strabismus (eye misalignment), affecting around 2-4 per cent of people, can lead to a loss of binocular vision and depth perception. This condition is one of the earliest recorded genetic disorders. More than 2,400 years ago, Hippocrates noted that children of parents with this trait also tended to show it. Indeed, some studies suggest around 30 per cent of individuals with strabismus have a close relative with the condition, demonstrating the important role of genetics. A number of the world's most famous artists may have owed their talents, to some degree, to this condition. Rembrandt's divergent squint, evident in some of his self-portraits, has led to the suggestion that his visual condition may have contributed to his ability to translate a 3-dimensional world to a 2-dimensional canvas. Albrecht Durer, who is credited with formalising and refining linear perspective in

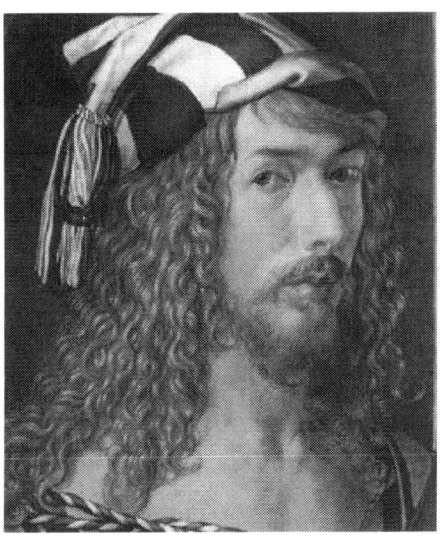

Albrecht Durer, self-portrait, 1498

Renaissance Art, is another artist who appeared to have suffered strabismus, evident from his self-portraits, as well as Leonard de Vinci and numerous others. It's worth looking to see how many self-portraits of well-known portrait artists appear to show they have strabismus.

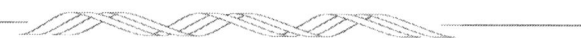

# HEARING & BALANCE DISORDERS

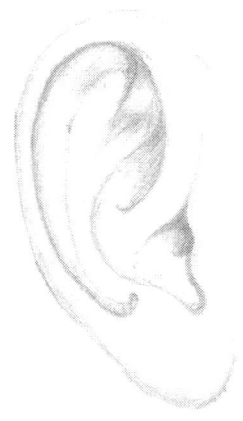

*What matters deafness of the ear, when the mind hears. The one true deafness, the incurable deafness, is that of the mind.*

Victor Hugo

Around 1 in 1,000 babies are born with a hearing impairment in the UK. Genetic factors account for as many as half of these cases with over 120 genes known to result in deafness when mutated. However, more than half of all recessively inherited cases of deafness result from mutations in just one gene, Connexin 26.

Around 4 per cent of the population carry a mutant Connexin 26 gene which normally produces a protein important in forming channels between cells to allow for the passage of small molecules and ions important in the inner ear. More severe disruptions of this same gene also lead to skin abnormalities. Individuals having only one copy of such a mutant gene tend to develop increasing skin thickness suggesting that a selective advantage could exist for this gene providing protection against possible cuts and infections, perhaps explaining why so many of the population still carry this gene variant. Another possible reason for the high frequency of this gene mutation, and other deafness-causing genes, is that many individuals with deafness marry another deaf person, some put the figure as high as 85 per cent. This is supported by the fact that 200 years ago Connexin 26 deafness was half as common. It was Alexander Graham Bell, whose mother and wife were both deaf, who speculated that continued intermarriage among the deaf would lead to increased numbers of deaf individuals prompting him to suggest closing residential schools for the deaf in favour of mainstream education.

Charles Darwin wrote in the *Origin of Species* that *"cats which are entirely white and have blue eyes are generally deaf"*. He then commented that *"this correlation was quite whimsical"*. However there are biological mechanisms linking albinism and deafness as melanin, the dark pigment found in the skin and the eyes, also has a function in the development in the ear. This can be seen in Waardeburg syndrome, a disorder that results from a number of mutations in certain genes involved in the function and development of pigment-producing cells, melanocytes. Accounting for around 1 per cent of all deaf individuals, this autosomal dominant disease is characterised by very pale blue eyes, changes in pigmentation of the hair, skin, and eyes that can often include a distinctive hair colouring such as a patch of white hair as well as hearing loss.

In addition to single gene defects affecting only deafness there also nearly 400 syndromes in which deafness is a feature, for example, Waardenburg Syndrome. There are also numerous other disorders that can lead to deafness in later life. Ludwig Van Beethoven produced some of his greatest works, such as *Ode to Joy* in 1824, after he became totally deaf. It was at around the age of thirty that he began to suffer from buzzing in both ears. Sometimes this would clear for a few months at a time but it eventually ended in complete

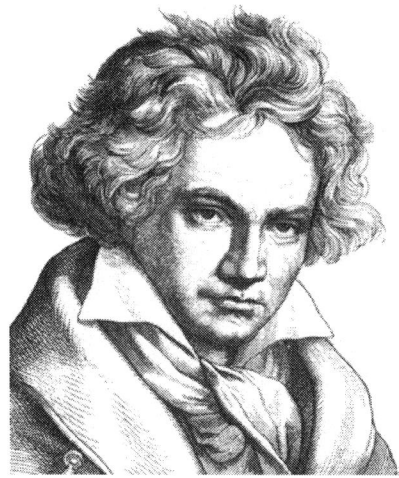

Ludwig van Beethoven by Emil Eugen Sachse, 1854

deafness. His autopsy in 1827 revealed abnormal growth of bone in the inner ear. One of the most important causes of chronic progressive hearing loss in adults is otosclerosis, a condition in which there is an abnormal growth of the tiny bones deep inside the ear which vibrate from sound waves. Beethoven's other bones also continued to overgrow in his head leading to a prominent forehead, enlarged jaw, and protruding chin. There are several other musicians and singers who have suffered from deafness due to otosclerosis, including Dina Carroll and Frankie Valli of the *Four Seasons*.

In 1856 a girl by the name of Steinin, at the Leipzig School for the Deaf, suddenly collapsed and died while being publicly told off by the headmaster for a misdemeanour. When the parents were informed it emerged that two of the girl's deaf brothers had also previously died following episodes of emotional stress. This autosomal recessive inherited disorder, now known as Jervell and Lange-Nielsen syndrome, is often the main suspect in the rare cases of sudden death among deaf individuals. It results from defects in a gene producing a protein involved in potassium ion channels, which in addition to the ear, are also important for heart muscles.

There are about 24,000 people in the UK who are both deaf and blind. Though, the majority of affected individuals lose their senses later in life from infections such as rubella, the major genetic cause for deaf-blindness is Usher syndrome. This results from mutations in a number of different genes playing roles in the development of the inner ear and retina. Children who inherit this autosomal recessive disorder lose their hearing and vision either very early, during the first decade of life, or later in adulthood depending on the genes involved. One well-known case of Usher syndrome was John Tracy, the son of the American actor Spencer Tracy and his wife Louise. They first noticed his deafness when a slamming door failed to wake him up at 10 months of age; he then lost his eyesight later in life. It was through their son that his parents founded the John Tracy Clinic in 1942, a private, non-profit education centre for infants and preschool children with hearing loss in Los Angeles. Rebecca Alexander has written an inspiring book, *Not Fade Away: A Memoir of Senses Lost and Found* in 2015, chronicling her battle with the disorder that has led to her, and her twin brother, gradually losing their sight and hearing from their early teens until the age of 30.

The Spanish painter Fransisco Goya became permanently deaf in 1792. In addition to his hearing loss, he also suffered problems with balance and coordination. This may have been due to an autoimmune disorder known as Vogt-Koyanagi-Harada that disrupts the workings of the inner ear. As well as hearing, the inner ear is also important for the detection of orientation and movement. Isolated from others by his deafness, he became increasingly occupied with the fantasies and inventions of his imagination and it has been

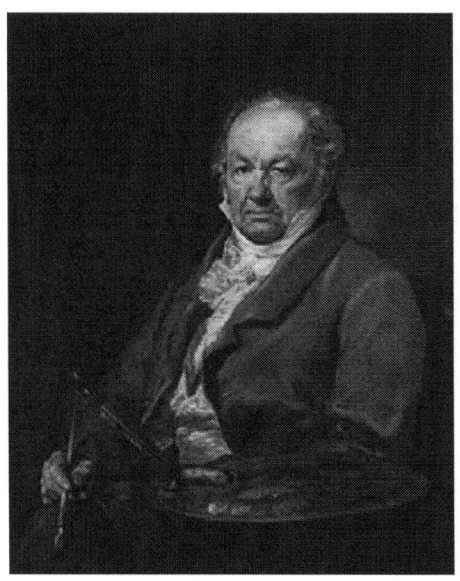

Francisco Goya by Vicente López Portaña, c. 1826

suggested that the haunting themes of Goya's "Black Paintings", created in the later years of his life, were influenced by his disease.

The balance organs in the inner ear consist of tubes and cavities containing fluid and small hairs which are moved in response to motion of the head. Spinning around can cause the fluid to keep sloshing around long after motion has ceased, with the hair cells still informing the brain that the body is moving, even after it has stopped – this causes the dizziness and nausea (Gr. *naus*, ship). A similar situation can occur whilst reading in a moving car – the inner ear senses the movement of the vehicle, but the eyes see only the book which is not moving. The resulting sensory conflict can lead to the typical symptoms of motion sickness,

One of the major conditions affecting the inner ear and leading to vertigo is Ménière's disease in which an excess of fluid in the inner ear causes swelling of the tubes and cavities. This disease was often considered to be sporadic, but over half of cases report other family members with the disorder, suggesting some genetic component. The author of *Gulliver's Travels*, Jonathan Swift suffered most of his life from periodic bouts of deafness, sometimes combined with illness or giddiness. He described rarely feeling safe from attacks of vertigo or from a deafening sound like rushing water in his ears that blocked out human voices. This worsened as he grew older, which, possibly in conjunction with Alzheimer's

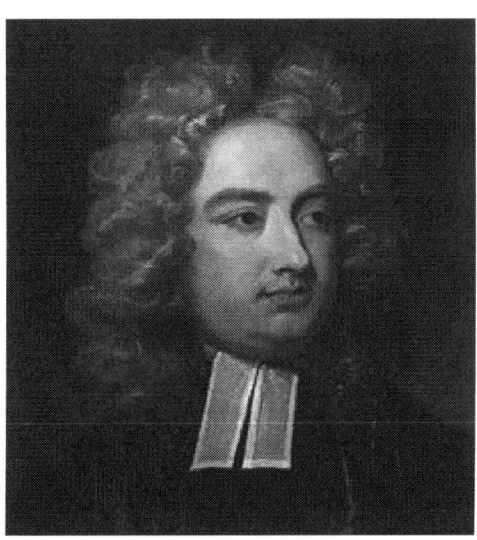

Jonathan Swift by Charles Jervas, 1870

disease, led to him being declared of unsound mind three years before his death in 1742. Swift had predicted his mental decay when he was in his 50s telling the poet Edward Young when they were gazing at the withered crown of a tree: *'I shall be like that tree; I shall die from the top*'. A number of other high-profile people also appear to have suffered from this condition. Martin Luther often wrote about the distress of vertigo, suspecting Satan to be the cause while Marilyn Monroe was known to experience vertigo and hearing problems.

Joubert's Syndrome is caused by mutations in a number of different genes resulting in the underdevelopment of the cerebellum, a small part of the lower portion of the brain important for coordinating movements. The British film-maker Andrew Kötting's documentary-style movie, *Gallivant* (1996), records a journey he took clockwise around the coast of Britain accompanied by his eight-year-old daughter Eden, who suffers from the disorder. Premiered to great acclaim at the Edinburgh Film Festival, it won the Channel 4 Best New Director prize thus raising awareness of this medical condition.

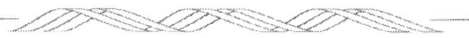

# PERIPHERAL NERVOUS SYSTEM

# DISORDERS

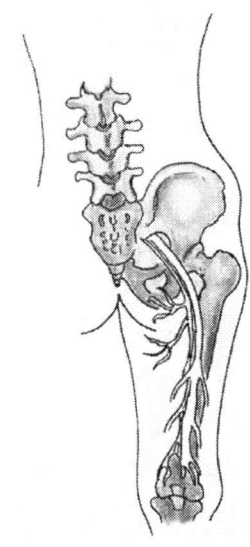

*If I'm out in public, I grab on to some charming, darling fellow who can steady me. I've been encouraged by the many men who have offered me their shoulders and arms.*

Julie Newmar

The nervous system has two distinct parts: the central nervous system consisting of the brain and spinal cord, and the peripheral nervous system describing the nerves outside the brain and spinal cord. Peripheral neuropathies are disorders involving the peripheral nerves such as sensory nerves responsible for transmitting sensations, such as pain and touch, motor nerves responsible for controlling muscle, and autonomic nerves that regulate automatic functions of the body, such as blood pressure. If motor neurons are damaged

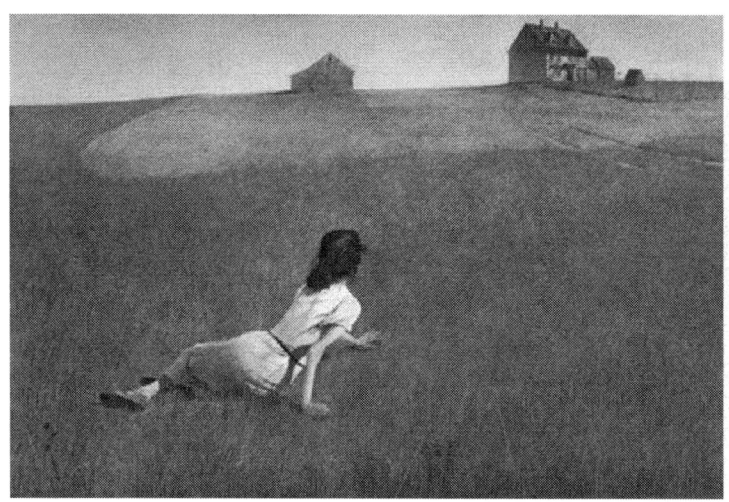

*Christina's World* (1948) by Andrew Wyeth

muscles may weaken or become paralysed. If sensory nerves are damaged, sensation may be lost or abnormal sensations may be felt.

The American painter Andrew Wyeth, when looking through his window, was captivated by the sight of a neighbour, picking blueberries while crawling through a field. *Christina's World* became one of the most recognised images in American art. Anna Christina Olson, the subject of the painting, lost the use of legs in her early 30s and it is thought she suffered from Charcot–Marie–Tooth disease. This is the most common hereditary motor and sensory neuropathy and is named after the three doctors who described the disorder in the early 20th century. Affecting around 1 in 2,500 people, this disorder usually results from damage of the membrane surrounding neuronal axons, known as the myelin sheath. Composed of fatty substances known as lipids, myelin can be likened to the insulation around an electrical wire, acting as an insulator to electrical signals, enabling nerve impulses to travel quickly. In demyelinating diseases, these myelin sheaths become degraded slowing the transport of impulses that would normally travel around 225 miles an hour. The loss of myelin leads to a slow progressive degeneration of muscles in the feet and lower legs which can spread to the hands and forearms, and generally presents in early adulthood. A number of mutations in different genes affecting the development and maintenance of myelin in the peripheral nerves can produce this condition. Todd MacCulloch retired from playing basketball with the Philadelphia 76ers in 2003 after he

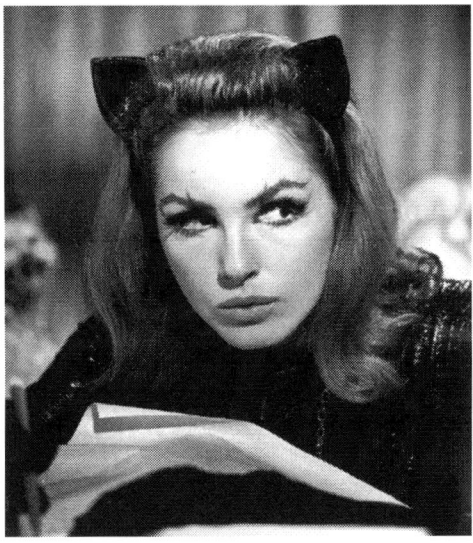

Julie Newmar, 1966

had been diagnosed with this condition which had been slowly reducing his physical strength, starting with numbness and tingling in his feet and then spreading to his hands. He now works as a commentator. Julie Newmar the American actress, dancer and singer, most famous for her role as *Cat Woman* in the *Batman* television series was diagnosed with the disorder in 2000 aged 67 after finding it increasingly difficult to walk and keep her balance.

The most common disease associated with a loss of myelin is multiple sclerosis. In this disorder, myelin is destroyed by the body's own immune system possibly in response to

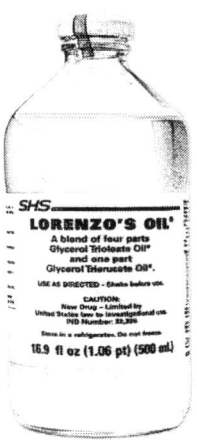

Lorenzo's oil

a combination of some environmental triggers and some degree of genetic susceptibility. One of the most common inherited myelin diseases is adrenoleukodystrophy. This results from defects in a gene that codes for an enzyme needed to break down Very Long Chain Fatty Acids that then build up in the brain killing neurons. Occurring in early life, children that have previously developed normally, quickly lose their sight, hearing, speech and movement. The film *Lorenzo's Oil* is based on the true story of Augusto and Michaela Odone, two parents in a relentless search for a cure for their son Lorenzo who was born in 1984 with the condition that had only been identified 10 years earlier. With no science backgrounds, they quickly set about learning everything possible about the disease and eventually developed a treatment that seemed to prevent it from progressing any further in their child. For this, Augusto Odone received an honorary PhD. Known as Lorenzo's Oil, it is a mixture of two fatty acids that in some studies prevents the build-up of Very Long Chain Fatty Acids in the body. Outliving his expected life expectancy by two decades

Lorenzo died in 2008 at the age of 30. However, the patent money from the oil continues to support an international research enterprise founded by the Odone's called the Myelin Project. Other mutations in the same gene causing adrenoleukodystrophy result in a related disorder known as adrenomyeloneuropathy, that has an adult-onset, typically between the ages of 20 and 30 years old. The Chilean musician Sebastian Santa Maria was diagnosed with this disorder at the age of 34, while he was working on the recording of his first solo album *Latino*, and died 3 years later in 1996. His brother Julio had also suffered and died from this same inherited disease aged 19.

A progressive loss in coordination can result from degeneration of neurons in the cerebellum of the brain and nerve tissue in the spinal cord, important for controlling muscle movement in the arms and legs. This can lead to the development of clumsy or awkward movements and unsteadiness, known as ataxia (Lat. *a*, lack of; *taxis*, order/coordination). Affecting around 1 in 50,000 people, the most common recessively inherited ataxia is Friedrich's ataxia resulting from mutations in a gene coding for a protein involved in mitochondria function. When this is disrupted, nerve cells of the spinal cord are unable to inefficiently use cellular energy leading to their degeneration. This disorder is relatively common among French Canadians with many inheriting the mutant gene from a couple, Jean Guyon and Mathurine Robin, both of whom emigrated from Normandy in 1634. The renowned British logician, Philip Edward Bertrand Jourdain, began to experience difficulties in walking as a young boy suffering from this same inherited disease as one of his sisters. By the time he became a student at Cambridge University he was unable to walk unaided. While many sufferers do not survive past their twenties, Jourdain lived just short of his 40th birthday, dying in 1919.

There are other forms of spinocerebellar ataxia that are dominantly inherited. These are caused by mutations in different genes encoding proteins found in nerve cells of the cerebellum and spinal cord. One of these genes is found in the family tree of President Abraham Lincoln. Either Captain Abraham Lincoln or Bathsheba Herring must have had

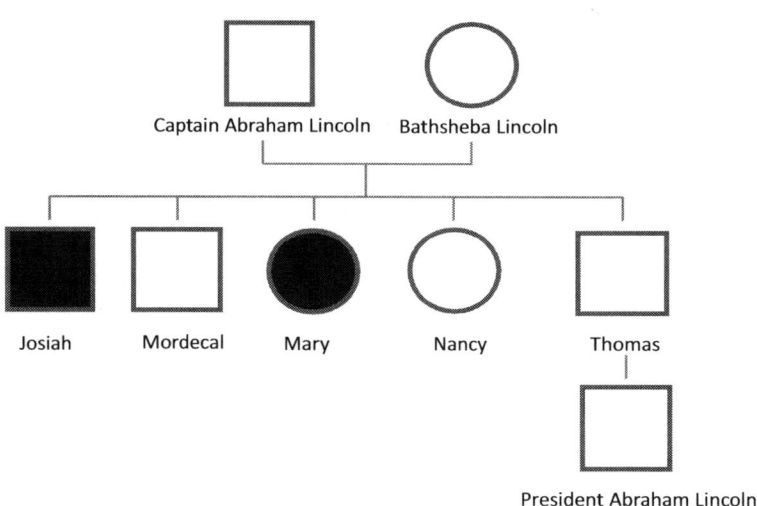

Part of the family tree of Abraham Lincoln showing affected individuals (shaded)

the affected gene and passed it on to at least two of their five children who subsequently suffered from the condition, and passed it on to a further ten generations. President Lincoln would have had a 25 per cent chance of inheriting the gene. As some of the other affected members of his family only developed symptoms as late as 68 years of age it could be possible that he himself had inherited the gene but had yet to show any symptoms by the time of his assassination at the age of 56.

# CENTRAL NERVOUS SYSTEM

# DISORDERS

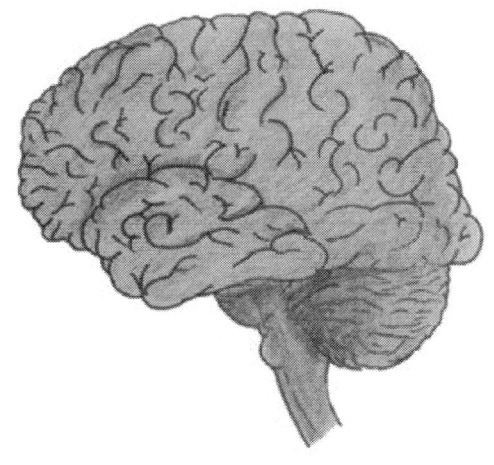

*A man who views the world the same at fifty as he did at twenty has wasted thirty years of his life.*

Muhammad Ali

The human brain, consists of about 100 billion neurons making around 100 trillion connections. These control our thoughts, memory, emotions, touch, motor skills, vision, breathing, temperature, hunger, and every process that regulates our body. Different

247

regions of the brain have different functions and different disorders of the brain affecting different regions lead to different symptoms. Different disorders may affect the brain at specific stages of life. Neurodevelopmental disorders such as autism, depression and schizophrenia first appear in early childhood, teens, or early adulthood, although their origins may lie much earlier in life. As we age, we become increasingly susceptible to neurodegenerative diseases such as Alzheimer's disease or Parkinson's disease.

Neurodevelopmental disorders result from a disruption in the development of the brain which can result from environmental and genetic factors and includes rare genetic syndromes as well as common, heritable conditions such as intellectual disability, autism, schizophrenia and major depression.

Autism spectrum disorder (ASD) is a condition that appears early in childhood development, and covers a range of conditions, including Asperger syndrome, that varies in severity, and are characterised by impaired social skills, communication problems, and repetitive behaviours. Those with lower levels of severity may need lesser support than those with more severe symptoms. Around 1 per cent of all children are diagnosed with ASD and it is more common in males than females. Changes in over 1,000 genes have been reported to be associated with ASD, many involved in brain development. However, not all people with these gene variations will be affected as most gene variations have only a small effect, and variations in many genes can combine with various environmental risk factors, to determine an individual's risk of developing this complex condition.

Some interesting studies investigating characteristic personality and behavioural traits linked to autism in the general population, often find higher levels in those working in science, technology, engineering or mathematics. Some studies have found an association between autism and first-degree relatives of mathematicians suggesting genetic links. Isaac Newton hardly spoke, was so engrossed in his work that he often forgot to eat, and was lukewarm or bad-tempered with the few friends he had. If no one turned up to his lectures, he gave them anyway, talking to an empty room. He had a nervous breakdown at 50 years of age, brought on by depression and paranoia. As a child, Einstein was also a loner, a late talker and repeated sentences obsessively until he was 7 years old. He also became notorious for giving confusing lectures, and he never felt comfortable delivering speeches, making small talk with people, or mingling with people. He was often forgetful of everyday items such as keys, and he quickly became known as the stereotypical 'absent-minded professor'.

Among those with autism, possibly around 1 per cent demonstrate certain abilities far in excess of average, often related to memory. For example, they may show exceptional puzzle skills, mathematical abilities and artistic or musical talents. This is known as savant syndrome with some studies suggesting a degree of genetic relatedness with autism. Stephen Wiltshire is a British architectural artist known for his amazing ability to draw a panoramic

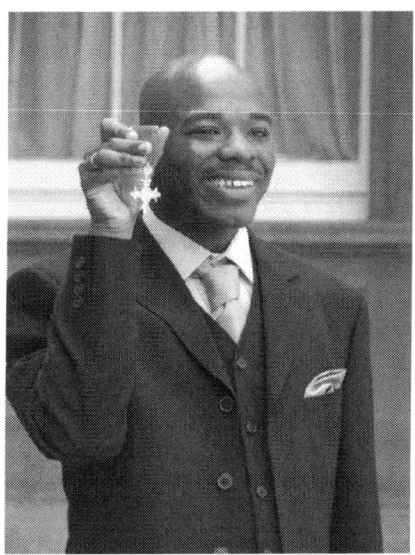

Stephen Wiltshire receiving an MBE for services to art in 2006

landscape from memory after seeing it just once. Diagnosed with autism at the age of 3, he was not able to speak fully until the age of 9. In 2011, following a 20-minute helicopter ride over New York city he drew a perfect 19ft long panorama of the whole city from memory alone.

Schizophrenia is a psychosis, which means that it affects a person's thinking, sense of self, and perceptions. Symptoms typically become evident during late adolescence or early adulthood which can include false perceptions such as hallucinations that can involve visual, auditory, olfactory, or tactile sensations. Delusions can also develop such that affected individuals may think they or someone else is being plotted against or controlled by others. Disordered thinking, impaired concentration, inappropriate emotional responses, erratic speech and behaviour, and difficulty with personal hygiene and everyday tasks can also be typical. Schizophrenia is as common as ASD affecting around 1 per cent of individuals. Though the risk of developing schizophrenia is only slightly higher for family members of affected individuals, studies in twins show there is a major genetic component. It seems variations in many genes contribute to the risk of developing schizophrenia and similar to autism spectrum disorder, it is thought multiple genetic changes, each with a small effect, combine with various environmental risk factors to increase the risk of developing this disorder. These environmental factors include early exposures to infections or severe stress. Recreational drugs such as cannabis, cocaine or LSD may also trigger symptoms of schizophrenia in people who are susceptible. This is suggested to have affected the charismatic frontmen and founders of two of the most influential bands. Both Syd Barrett, of *Pink Floyd*, and Peter Green of *Fleetwood Mac* left their respective bands and were subsequently diagnosed with schizophrenia, possibly resulting from the taking of psychedelic drugs. Though Peter Green continued to play, Syd Barrett became a recluse and died alone aged 60.

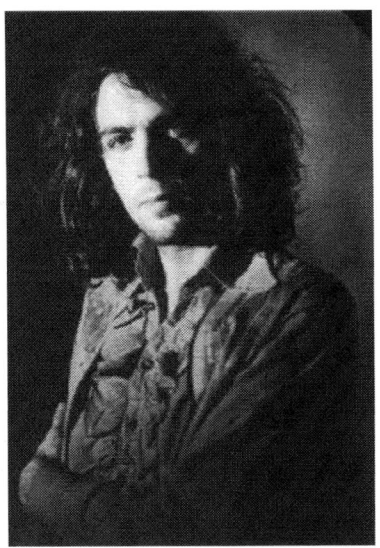

Syd Barrett, 1969

Depression is a disorder that affects mood, behaviour, and health. It commonly begins in late adolescence or early adulthood, although it can appear at any age. Affected individuals may have difficulty functioning in their daily lives and also have a higher risk of substance abuse problems and dying by suicide. Suicide is the leading cause of death among young people aged 20-34 years in the UK. Depression is known to run in families, suggesting the existence of genetic factors, and similarly to neurodevelopmental disorders, it seems that variations in many genes, each with a small effect, combine to increase the risk of developing depression. Some of these genes may control the activity of chemicals called neurotransmitters, which relay chemical signals to allow neurons to communicate with one another. Environmental factors, such as stress, are also very important.

As a possible example of a level of heritability in depression, the comedian Ben

Stiller has said he has a 'rich history of bipolar manic depression' in his family. In addition to himself, his actor-comedian parents, Jerry Stiller and Anne Meara, have both suffered and his maternal grandmother committed suicide. A co-star in many of his movies, Owen Wilson has also battled the disease with a suicide attempt in 2007. It appears many comedians struggle with depression, and importantly many, together with other prominent members of society, are discussing the issue and breaking taboos. When Prince Harry first

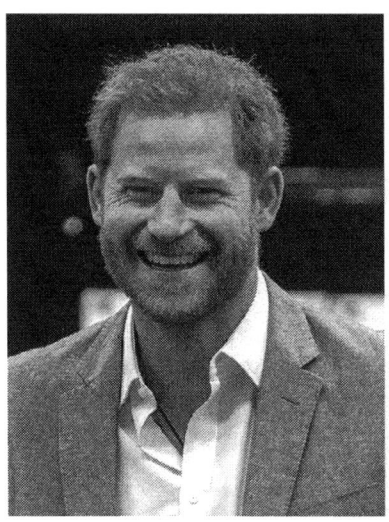

Prince Harry, 2019

opened up about his mental health issues, some medical experts commented that he had probably done more for communicating such diseases in his first 25-minute interview then they had been able to do in their whole careers.

Around 2.5 per cent of people in the UK have an intellectual disability. This is defined as a reduced intellectual ability and difficulty with everyday activities such as household tasks, socialising or managing money, that affects someone over their entire life. Learning disabilities together with dyslexia, dyscalculia and autism, affect up to 10 per cent of the population. The two most common genetic causes of intellectual disabilities are Down syndrome and Fragile X syndrome.

Fragile X syndrome affects around 1 in 4,000 males, varying in severity from mild to severe mental retardation with physical characteristics such as an elongated face and large or protruding ears. It results from mutations in a gene on the X chromosome, required for normal neural development; hence this X-inherited disease tends to more severely affect males than females. The type of mutation in this particular disorder is known as a trinucleotide repeat expansion where various numbers of a repeat CGG sequence occur in a gene; less than 50 times in unaffected and over 200 times in affected individuals.

The most common neurodegenerative disease and the most common cause of dementia (Lat. *de*; away; *mentis*; mind) is Alzheimer's disease. This results from the degeneration of tissue in certain areas of the brain leading to a progressive deterioration in mental function. This disease also associates with the accumulation of clumps of amyloid protein, called plaques, and the accumulation of tau protein as tangles. The aggregation of proteins in the brain are a hallmark of many different neurodegenerative disorders. For example, tau accumulation in different regions of the brain such as in the frontal and temporal lobes causes frontotemporal dementia leading to behavioural abnormalities rather than memory loss while progressive supranuclear palsy results from such aggregations in the midbrain. Accumulation of a protein in aggregates called Lewy bodies are found in Parkinson's disease and Lewy body dementia, while protein aggregates also appear in Huntington's disease and Prion diseases.

While the causes of Alzheimer's are still not precisely understood, genetic factors are implicated in familial and early-onset cases, which account for around 7% of all

Alzheimer's. Early-onset describes the occurrence of the disease in individuals under the age of 65. The best-selling British author Terry Pratchett suffered a form of early-onset disease, diagnosed at the age of 59. Late-onset cases also have some genetic components with studies suggesting there is a higher chance in relatives of those affected with Alzheimer's disease then there would be in the general population. Nevertheless, the only gene implicated so far is the APOE gene coding for a protein involved in the transport of lipids and in the metabolism of cholesterol.

One of the first effects of Alzheimer's disease is the gradual loss of short-term memory and the ability to reason and concentrate. The British Prime Minister, Harold Wilson, first noticed these effects while still in office at the age of 60. A doctor recorded that while his memory of years gone remained excellent, he could not remember what he had

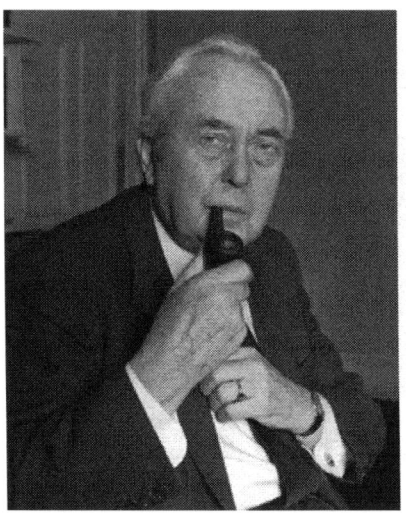

Harold Wilson, 1969

had for breakfast on the same day. It may have been the realisation of this and the experience of seeing the mental decline of his mother who also died from the disease, that could have prompted his unexpected resignation in 1976. President Ronald Reagan made his diagnosis of Alzheimer's disease public in 1994, but it was some years earlier, while he was in his second term of office, that some psychologists began to detect possible signs of the disorder in his conversation, speech and behaviour. At one press conference, he was asked about his plans for talks with the Russians on space weapons. He seemed confused by the question and was unable initially to find the words. Nancy Reagan whispered loudly, "Tell them we're doing everything we can". "We're doing everything we can," he echoed. Remarkably, despite his growing dementia, he is remembered chiefly for his astute handling of the cold war, often against general advice. After he left office, the disease went on to slowly ravage his mental capacity until he died of pneumonia in 2004. Infection is one of the most common cause of death in dementia patients, particularly pneumonia, as impaired swallowing allows food or drink to enter the lungs, where an infection can begin.

British actor and comedian Dudley Moore, also an accomplished pianist, first noticed problems with the co-ordination of his finger movements while playing. Later he would find it difficult to remember his lines, his speech started to slur and had problems maintaining his balance. In 1995 he was fired by Bette Miller from his final film *The Mirror*

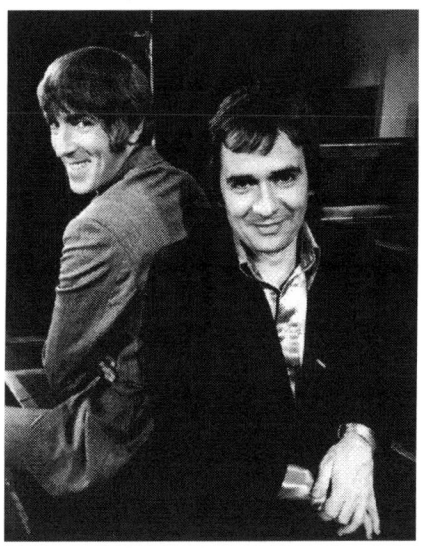

Dudley Moore (right) and Peter Cook, 1974

*Has Two Faces* as he was unable to remember his lines. At first, misinterpreted by many as a sign of drunkenness, he was finally diagnosed with the neurodegenerative disease known as progressive supranuclear palsy in 1997. Though showing only a low degree of inheritance, progressive supranuclear palsy may result from mutations in the gene for tau leading to the protein aggregating in the midbrain. This brain region is important in balance and eye-movements. One of the earliest tell-tale signs Dudley Moore had was an inability to control movements of the eye, particularly vertical eye movements sometimes referred to as "dirty-tie syndrome" as those affected cannot see that they are dropping food when they eat. This later progressed into more severe vision and balance problems and dementia. Shortly before his death, aged 66 years old in 2002, he set up the Dudley Moore Research Fund, raising awareness and generating funds for research in finding a cure for this disease

Robin Williams, like Dudley Moore, found he was struggling to remember lines, particularly during the filming of *Night at the Museum 3*. This developed into a bewildering array of other symptoms starting with insomnia, constipation, and an impaired sense of

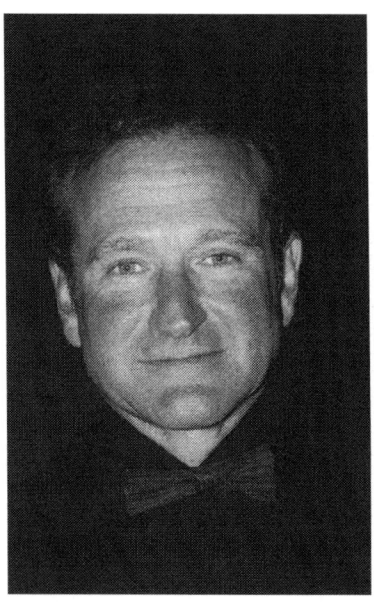

Robin Williams, 2001

smell that soon spiralled into extreme anxiety, tremors, and difficulty in reasoning. He also found it difficult to judge distances, bruising himself walking into doors and he would wake at night with delusions and paranoia. For nearly a year, he tried to find out what was wrong with him, talking about the need to "reboot his brain". Later, symptoms similar to Parkinson's disease emerged, including a weakening of the voice and a hand tremor leading doctors to diagnose him with Parkinson's disease in the months before he died. However, he was convinced it was something else and sadly committed suicide in 2014 aged 63. His autopsy results later showed he had suffered from a severe type of dementia known as Lewy body dementia. Making up around 10-15 per cent of all diagnosed dementia, Lewy body dementia is characterised by both dementia and Parkinson's disease symptoms. Individuals often also have vivid hallucinations, particularly at night, fluctuating cognition, and sleep disruption. They may also lose their sense of smell - a symptom also common in Parkinson's and Alzheimer's diseases. Like Alzheimer's disease and progressive supranuclear palsy, it is caused by the accumulation of protein aggregates in the brain. However, in this disease the protein aggregates are called Lewy bodies and consist of the protein alpha-synuclein.

Two well-known writers whose work appears to have been affected by their encroaching Lewy body dementia are the Prussian philosopher Immanuel Kant and the British artist, poet and playwright, Mervyn Peake. Immanuel Kant showed clear symptoms of dementia, memory loss, repetitive behaviours such as constantly buttoning and unbuttoning his clothes, fluctuations in his mental abilities and hallucinations. Mervyn Peake's sketches during his illness portrayed the visual hallucinations he was experiencing while paranoid delusions become apparent in his later poetry. It is speculated that Charles Dickens may have based the character *Ebenezer Scrooge* who was visited by ghosts in the night, on someone with Lewy body dementia who was experiencing night-time hallucinations.

Parkinson's disease affects around 1 in 500 people and results from the loss of neurons in a part of the brain controlling muscle movement. These neurons make a chemical neurotransmitter called dopamine which sends signals to coordinate movements. In a similar way to Lewy body dementia, aggregates of a protein, alpha-synuclein, builds up in these cells killing them - but in a different part of the brain. This affects physical movement leading to tremor, slowness of movement and muscle stiffness or rigidity. For around 15 per cent of patients, there is some family history of the disease but the extent to which this is a result of shared genes rather than shared environmental risk is still uncertain. However, in the same way as Alzheimer's disease, genetic factors appear to be more predominant when the disease begins earlier in life. Several genes have been found in early-onset Parkinson's disease, in which development of symptoms begin at around the ages of 40 and 50 years or younger and tend to be inherited recessively. These include the previously mentioned tau gene and the alpha-synuclein gene that is also involved in Lewy body dementia.

One prominent sufferer of early-onset Parkinson's disease is Michael J. Fox who first noticed symptoms at the young age of 29 whilst working on movie *Doc Hollywood*. He awoke one morning in 1990 with a persistent tremor of his left little finger which then progressed to other areas of his body before he was diagnosed a year later. He now focuses much of his energy on his Michael J. Fox Foundation for Parkinson's Research which has raised much awareness and contributed many millions of dollars for research into the disorder.

Ozzy Osbourne has suffered from tremors for many years, first noticing them in his 20s and thinking they might be to do with his drinking. Then in 2003, he was diagnosed

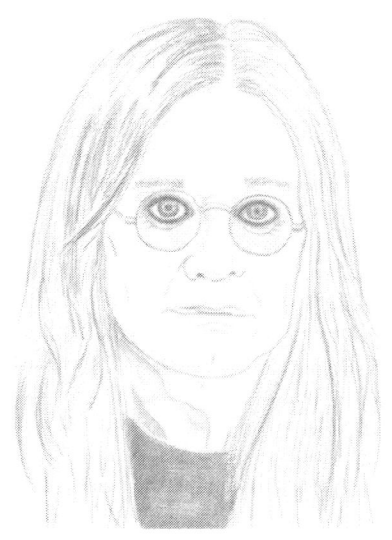

Ozzy Osboune

with Parkin disease. This results from mutations in a gene, called parkin leading to a disorder similar to Parkinson's disease. Though sharing many clinical features with Parkinson's, though with a slower progression, Parkin disease is pathologically very different to Parkinson's disease as affected brains do not contain the typical protein deposits seen in Parkinson's. *"I'd always assumed it was the booze and stuff,"* he explained, *"Now I've found it all stems from the family. When I told my sister she said, 'Not you as well? Mum had that and Auntie Elsie and your grandma.' I'm like, 'Thanks for f\*\*king telling me'. Me walking around thinking I've got some drug paralysis."* In early 2020 he told the public about his diagnosis and the medication he takes to combat the involuntary tremors; this is usually a form of dopamine, the neurotransmitter that is decreased in both this disease and Parkinson's disease.

Parkinson's disease has possibly played a major role in events of the last century by affecting a number of former dictators. It is likely that the disease was a key factor in Adolf Hitler's downfall. He first began to show symptoms in 1934 with newsreels showing tremors in his hand and a shuffling walk. As with so many governments, his medical condition was kept secret and by the time of the Normandy landings, he had suffered from the disease for

10 years and had in addition developed cognitive problems suggestive of dementia. Around a third of Parkinson's suffers also develop dementia. However, Hitler would not be the last European fascist dictator to succumb to the effects of Parkinson's disease. Francisco Franco was diagnosed with the disease in the 1960s and spent his last six years of rule in a highly weakened, often bed-ridden, state. Parkinson's disease, or possibly motor neuron disease, has also been implicated in the death of the Chinese dictator, Mao Zedong in 1975. His successor Deng Xiaoping also suffered from the disease. Both men continued to rule for several years whilst being plagued with the symptoms.

One day in the 1950s the wife of Woody Guthrie, the famous American folk singer, noticed her husband walking lopsidedly. This was soon followed by slurred speech and uncontrollable rages. Eventually, he lost all ability to talk, read, or walk and the only way he could communicate with his wife and children was by waving his arm at cards printed with the words 'Yes' and No'. In 1967 he died from the disease, which had previously killed his mother, from whom he had inherited it.

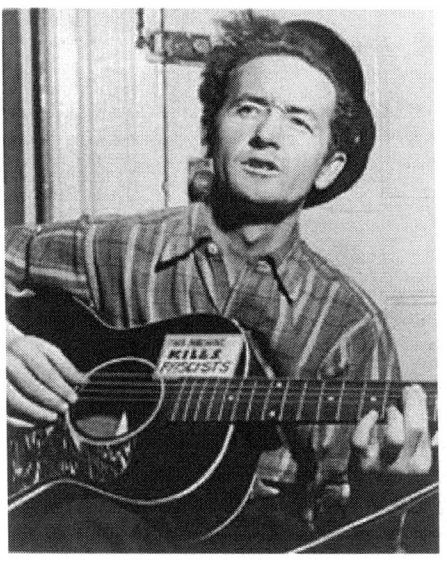

Woodie Guthrie, 1943

Huntington's disease, often referred to as "Woody Guthrie's disease" in the U.S, is an autosomal dominantly inherited disorder affecting around 1 in 20,000 individuals. It is caused by a mutation resulting in an altered protein that clumps together inside neurons killing these cells. This particularly affects neurons in brain areas responsible for mental abilities and movement coordination leading to the gradual development of abnormal movements and changes in cognition, behaviour, and personality. With an onset of symptoms usually between the ages of 30 and 50, a persons' ability to walk, think, talk and reason progressively diminish until death.

As the disease is inherited in an autosomal dominant fashion a parent with Huntington's disease has a 50 per cent chance of passing it on to any of their children. Their children have to decide whether or not to have themselves tested for the presence of the mutant gene. Should the results prove positive they would live with the certainty of developing symptoms of the disease before the age of 50. Insurance companies now legally have the right to know the outcome of any such test.

Huntington's disease has been reported since the 16th century, through the Renaissance physician Paracelsus who used the term "*chorea*", the Greek word for dance, to describe the shaking and twitching that people with the disease went through. However, it was in 1872, that George Huntington, aged only 22, provided the first scientific description of the disease emphasising the hereditary nature of the disorder. The family he studied on Long Island were ancestors of a man by the name of Jeffrey Francis who emigrated from England, carrying the Huntington mutated gene, in 1634. English colonists in America called the disease Saint Vitus Dance (St Vitus is the patron saint of dancers), and many of the "witches" at the infamous Salem Witch Trials of 1692 in Massachusetts, are now believed to have had Huntington's disease; their uncontrollable, irregular, jerky movements and odd behaviour were seen as possession by the devil. Perhaps some of these may have been related to the same family described by George Huntington.

Prion diseases are rare infectious degenerative diseases of the brain characterised by massive neuronal death leaving open areas in the brain resembling a sponge – hence they are often known as transmissible spongiform encephalopathies. These diseases are caused by a protein that normally functions in cell signalling. However, this particular protein has the peculiar capacity to convert into an abnormal form called a prion (an acronym for proteinaceous infection) that can bind to each other to form aggregates that kill the cell. Strangely, this abnormal form of prion is infectious in that it causes normal prion proteins to convert to the abnormal form starting a cascade across cells leading to their deaths. These diseases can either be inherited, such as familial Creutzfeldt-Jakob disease (CJD), or acquired as in the variant CJD and kuru.

The symptoms of CJD are a rapidly progressive dementia and loss of coordinated movement, with death often occurring within six months of onset. George Balanchine, one

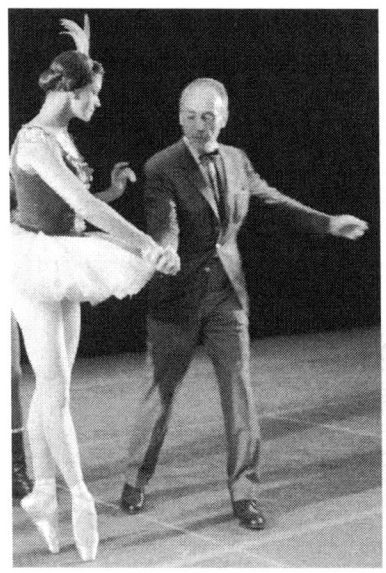

George Balanchine, 1963

of the 20th century's greatest choreographers, died of CJD, which was diagnosed after his death. The first signs appeared in 1978 when he began losing his balance while dancing, followed soon after by deterioration in eyesight and hearing until he became totally incapacitated. *"I'm finished. I can't hear, I walk like a drunken man"* he said, shortly before dying a few years after developing the first symptoms at the age of 79.

Another prion disease affects the thalamus part of the brain controlling sleep. Fatal familial insomnia was first described by an Italian country doctor, Ignazio Roiter, who married into a family suffering from this autosomal dominant condition. His wife's aunts both died after developing confusion, paranoia and remaining sleepless, vegetating in a dream-like state for the last months of their lives. He was able to trace the occurrence of the disease in his family over a period of more than 250 years.

Only a small percentage of prion disease cases run in families with most prion diseases developing sporadically in the absence of any mutation or as a result of infection with abnormally formed prion protein. This was first noted in the Fore tribe of Papua New Guinea in the 1950s. During funeral rituals, members of the tribe would eat the brains of dead relatives leading to the spread of a prion disease known as kuru, which means "trembling" in the language of the Fore. In a similar way, some cases of CJD in the U.S. have developed from the use of human growth hormone extracted from the pituitary glands of patients who died from CJD, though the known incidence of these cases is small and this procedure was discontinued in 1977. Another form of CJD, called "variant CJD", can be caused from consuming cows suffering from bovine spongiform encephalopathy (BSE), commonly called "mad cow disease". However, since the link between variant CJD and BSE was discovered in 1996, strict controls have proved very effective in preventing meat from infected cattle entering the food chain and the number of human cases are very low.

# GENES & CANCER

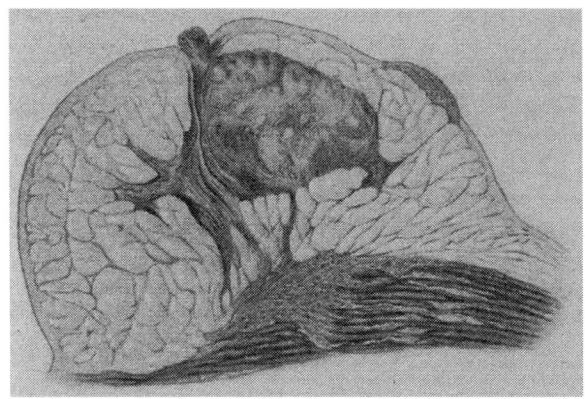

*Life comes with many challenges. The ones that should not scare us are the ones we can take on and take control of.*

Angelina Jolie

Hippocrates was one of the first to describe different kinds of cancers, using the word *oncos* (Gr. swelling) to describe benign tumours, and *carcinos* (Gr. crab) for malignant tumours possibly due to the appearance of the cut surface of some solid malignant tumours which

264

can vaguely resemble the silhouette of a crab. However, he was certainly not the first to document cancers. A papyrus dating to 1500 BC in ancient Egypt describes how breast cancers were treated by using a hot piece of metal to burn away the tissue.

Cancer describes an uncontrolled division of cells. These cells can then possibly invade nearby tissues and implant themselves into distant sites (known as metastasis). This unregulated cell growth is caused by damage to DNA, resulting in mutations to specific genes coding for proteins regulating cell growth and division, known as proto-oncogenes and tumour suppressor genes. Proto-oncogenes promote cell growth in a variety of ways by coding for proteins such as hormones, signal receptors, or transcription factor proteins which can increase expression of other genes. Tumour suppressor genes, on the other hand, code for anti-proliferation signals and proteins that suppress mitosis and cell growth. These tumour suppressors are normally activated by cell stress or DNA damage, thereby serving to halt cell division to carry out DNA repair, preventing mutations from being passed on to daughter cells.

In 1866, Paul Pierre Broca was the first to describe a family with a high incidence of breast and ovarian cancer. After his wife developed breast cancer while quite young, he traced the disorder going back four generations in her relatives and so demonstrating that it could be inherited. However, many scientists were sceptical of Broca's hereditary hypothesis at the time and so left cancer research and focused on neuroanatomy and is now remembered for the discovery of the "Broca's area", a region of the brain involved in organising language.

Familial cancer syndromes result from the inheritance of a mutation in a tumour suppressor gene or a proto-oncogene gene, that increases the chance of developing cells dividing uncontrollably and thus forming cancer. Mutations in tumour suppressor genes generally act in a recessive manner with a mutation in the second normal copy of the gene needed before a cell transforms into a cancer cell. For instance, individuals who inherit a mutation in a gene for p53 have an increased risk of developing a variety of cancers if they acquire mutations in their second copy of the p53. This is called Li-Fraumeni syndrome. Reza Dehghani, the founder of Criminal Clothing, died aged 32 in 2008, having suffered from cancer caused by inheriting the mutant gene for this disease. Neither his grandmother, his mother's sister, or his sister, who inherited the same gene defect lived through their 30s.

There are other examples of familial cancer syndromes. For example, mutations in the retinoblastoma gene increase an individual's risk of developing cancer of the eye retina. Mutations in BRCA1 or BRCA2 increase an individual's risk of developing breast and ovarian cancer, and von Hippel-Lindau syndrome associates with the development of various tumours, particularly in the adrenal glands.

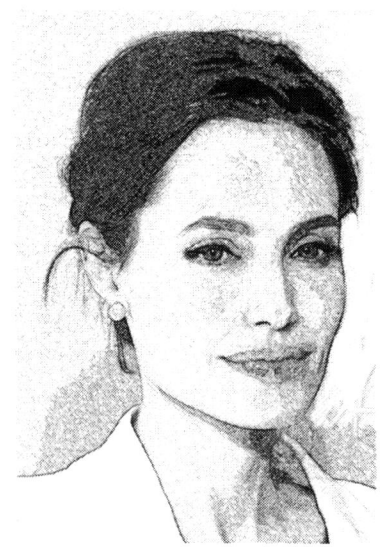

Angelina Jolie

The BRCA1 and BRCA2 genes are tumour suppressor genes producing proteins involved in repairing damaged DNA. Mutations in these genes lead to more DNA damage, to the point that other genes controlling cell growth and division also become unregulated leading to the development of cancer, particularly breast and ovarian. In 2013 Angelina Jolie, age 37 years old, underwent a preventive double mastectomy, followed later by removal of her ovaries and fallopian tubes, after learning she had an inherited a mutant BRCA1 gene. Her mother and grandmother died from ovarian cancer and her aunt from breast cancer. Following her operation, a global increase in BRCA gene testing occurred. But, in the US a company, Myriad Genetics, held a patent for the BRCA gene allowing them to charge $3000 for testing. Genes cannot be patented in other parts of the world. However, Angelia Jolie pushed for wider accessibility of BRCA gene testing and that helped to lead to a U.S. Supreme Court ruling in 2013, invalidating the patents and leading to a large reduction in the cost of testing. The "Angeline Jolie effect" on breast cancer awareness has almost doubled the levels of testing and preventative operations, in numerous countries including the UK, US and Australia.

Von Hippel-Lindau syndrome occurs due to mutations of the Von Hippel-Lindau tumour suppressor gene resulting in the growth of tumours in various parts of the body such as in the central nervous system, and particularly in the adrenal gland. It has been suggested that the hostility underlying the famous American Hatfield-McCoy feud of the late 1800s may have been partly due to the consequences of Von Hippel-Lindau disease. Generations of the two families fought often deadly battles over land, timber rights and even a pig and are the subject of dozens of books songs and countless jokes. It seems that the McCoy family was pre-disposed to bad tempers partly because many of them had adrenal gland tumours, which even now many of their descendants still suffer from. This tumour leads to increased production of adrenaline causing a tendency toward explosive tempers in addition to high blood pressure, pounding headaches, heart palpitations, facial flushing, nausea and vomiting.

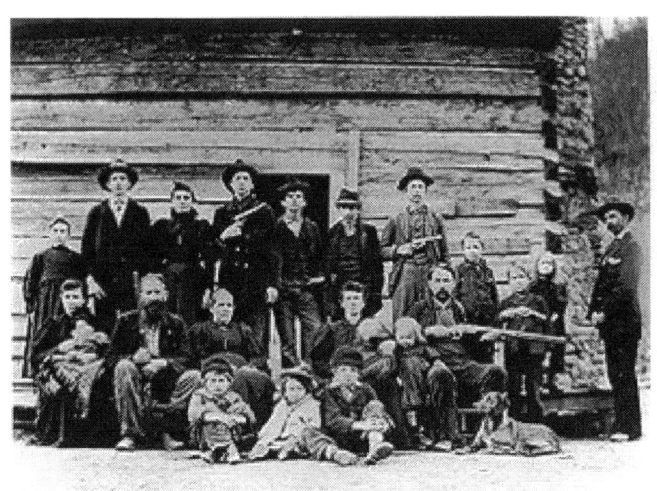

The Hatfield clan, 1887

The Philadelphia translocation is a specific chromosomal abnormality where parts of chromosomes 9 and 22 swap places resulting in the formation of a fused gene. This new abnormal gene interferes with the cell cycle speeding up cell division and disrupting the repair of DNA damage. This consequently results in an increased chance of developing chronic myelogenous leukaemia (CML). Kareem Abdul-Jabbar the retired American basketball player, coach, actor, and author announced that he was suffering from Philadelphia chromosome-positive chronic myeloid leukaemia in 2009, and was awarded the Double Helix Medal for his work in raising awareness of this disease and for promoting cancer research.

# DNA REPAR & PREMATURE AGEING

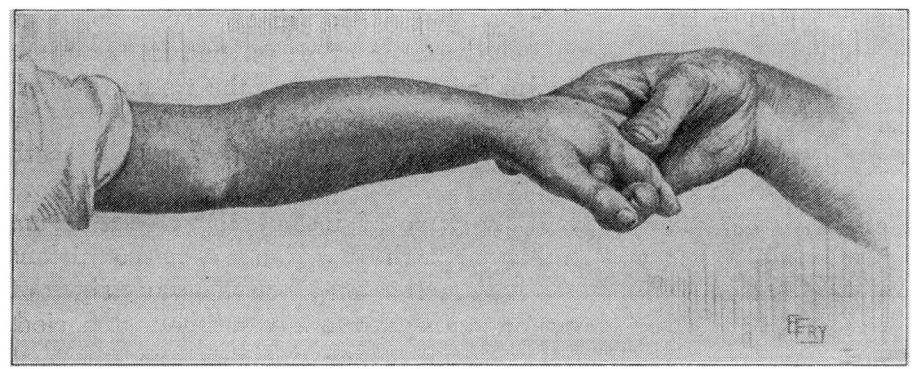

*DNA repair stands as the dike between us and the inundation of mutations.*

Robert Weinberg

An average cell normally acquires around 50,000 to 500,000 DNA damages per day. This occurs during normal metabolic processes inside the cell, but can also occur upon exposure to other sources of DNA damaging agents such as UV light. Whilst this constitutes only a tiny fraction of the human genome, a single unrepaired lesion to a critical cancer-related gene, as just described, can have drastic consequences. Therefore, DNA repair is an important process which constantly operates in cells. If the rate of DNA damage exceeds the capacity of the cell to repair it, the accumulation of errors can overwhelm the cell and result in cancer or cell death. Therefore, inherited diseases associated with faulty DNA repair result and an increased sensitivity to agents that can damage DNA. Diseases of this kind include xeroderma pigmentosum characterised by the development of multiple skin cancers and Werner syndrome that leads to premature ageing. More severe forms of accelerated ageing are called progeria.

Xeroderma pigmentosum results from an inability of the cells to repair UV damage to DNA, leading to the development of multiple skin cancers. Normally, DNA damage from UV light is repaired through a pathway where a damaged bit of DNA is replaced with the correct sequence from the opposing strand. In this disease, certain enzymes needed in this pathway are missing leading to DNA damage not being readily fixed. There are several types of xeroderma pigmentosum resulting from mutations of different genes that alter enzymes in this process. Naturally, the most important part of managing the condition is reducing exposure to the sun. An episode of an American series called *Extreme Makeover* involved the Pope family with a daughter Shelly who suffers from this disease; after the show, *Disney World* had a special night-time opening, midnight to 4 am, so that affected children could spend time at the amusement park.

In 1886, Dr Jonathan Hutchinson described a case of a 3-year-old boy who had features resembling those of an elderly man, leading to the term progeria (Gr. *pro*; early, *geras*; old age). Affecting around 1 in 8 million new-borns, this rare genetic condition leads to characteristics of accelerated ageing occurring from around the age of 2 years old with most sufferers dying in their early teens from heart disease or other age-related problems. While the disease can be dominantly inherited most cases result from a mutation occurring during the early stages of cell division in a newly conceived child or the gametes of one of the parents, known as a de novo mutation. It has been suggested that the American author F. Scott Fitzgerald could have been describing this disorder in his short novel *The curious case of Benjamin Button* published in 1921 about a child born with features of an elderly man.

*The Child Who's Older Than Her Grandmother* is a UK documentary first screened in 2005, telling the tragic story of Hayley Okines, a six-year-old girl born with progeria. A popular child at school, she put a lot of energy into raising awareness of the condition, including recording a song with the *Kids Choir 2000 for the Progeria Research Foundation*, before dying in 2015, aged 17. one of the oldest known persons with Progeria, surviving to the age of 26 before his death in June 2011, was Leon Botha, South African hip-hop artist and

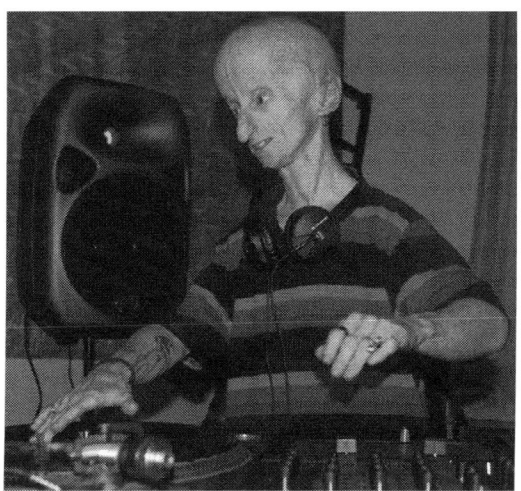

Leon Botha

painter. The increased atherosclerosis he suffered due to the disease lead to him undergoing heart bypass surgery, and he suffered a stroke some years later.

Another disorder characterised by accelerated ageing is Werner syndrome leading to a dramatic and rapid appearance of features associated with normal ageing. It is thought that the altered Werner protein interferes with the ability of cells to divide normally. Individuals with this disorder typically grow and develop normally until they reach puberty after which a premature ageing occurs involving greying and loss of hair, a hoarse voice, wrinkled skin, and the development of many disorders associated with ageing such as cataracts, skin ulcers, type 2 diabetes, atherosclerosis, osteoporosis and some types of cancer. In the 1996 movie *Jack*, Robin Williams plays a boy who is affected by Werner syndrome and is trying to live a normal life.

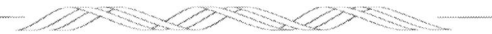

# DNA: PAST, PRESENT & FUTURE

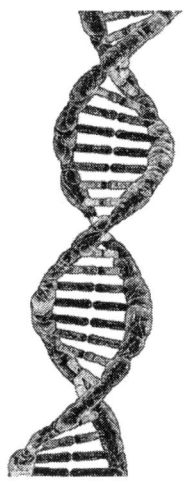

*It's lots of fun to blow bubbles but it's wiser to prick them yourself before someone else tries to.*

Oswald Avery

On April 25, 1953, James Watson and Francis Crick published an article in the journal *Nature* that revealed the structure of DNA. Often, the history of DNA is told as though it started with this discovery. However, the story began some time earlier.

In the second half of the 19th century, many fundamental concepts in biology were established as scientists began to study and understand cells. Matthias Schleiden and Theodor Schwann first showed that all tissues have a cellular origin and that animals and plants consist of cells. Louis Pasteur and Rudolph Virchow then demonstrated that new cells could only arise from other cells. This importantly disproved the previous notion of spontaneous generation; that new cells arise from lifeless matter. In parallel to these advances in cytology, the basic theories of heredity and evolution were being addressed with the publication of *On the Origin of the Species by Means of Natural Selection* in 1859 by Charles Darwin and Gregor Mendel's discovery of the laws of heredity in 1865.

Investigations to understand the molecular mechanisms underlying the basis of genetics then started to gain momentum. In 1866, Ernst Haeckel proposed that the nucleus contained the factors responsible for the transmission of hereditary traits and in the 1870s, Walter Flemming identified chromosomes within the nucleus. Using a red aniline dye to stain the cells of salamander embryos, he noticed red threads that differently distributed and doubled during cell division, naming these chromosomes (Gr. *Chrom*; coloured body) and calling the process of cell division, mitosis (Gr. *Mitos*; thread, referring to the spindly chromosomes). This allowed Theodor Boveri, in the late 1880s, to determine that chromosomes carry the genetic information in a cell.

The first person to isolate what we now know as DNA, or nucleic acid, was the Swiss scientist, Friedrich Miescher. His partial deafness prevented him from becoming a physician, and so he instead went to work in the lab of Felix Hoppe-Seyler at Schloss Hohentübingen, Germany, in 1868, who had just discovered the binding of oxygen to haemoglobin in red blood cells. Miescher was given the job over the next few years of trying to extract nuclei from white blood cells that he got from pus-filled bandages from a nearby hospital. Notoriously difficult to obtain, Miescher used different salt solutions followed by alkaline extraction and acidification. This resulted in a precipitate of a new compound being formed, that he called "nuclein" as it came from the nucleus. He was soon appointed professor of physiology in Basel at the young age of 28-years-old, though dying not long after, in 1885, of tuberculosis. His former teacher, C. Ludwig, wrote to him shortly before his death: *"I know what it is to give up well-loved, hopeful work. Sad as it is, there remains for you the satisfaction of having completed immortal studies in which the main point has been the knowledge of the nucleus; and so, as men work on the cell in the course of the following centuries, your name will be gratefully remembered as the pioneer of this field."* Following Miescher's departure from his lab, Hoppe-Seyler employed another scientist, Albrecht Kossel, who was able to determine that nuclein was comprised of four bases and sugar molecules (nucleotides) for which he won the Nobel Prize in Medicine.

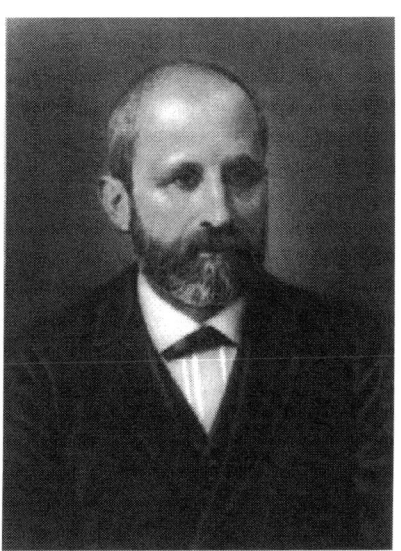

Fiedrich Miescher

In 1902, the British physician Archibald Garrod applied Mendel's laws of inheritance to a human disease publishing *The Incidence of Alkaptonuria: A Study of Chemical*

*Individuality*. By studying family histories of the disease, which results in the development of arthritis together with very dark urine, he was able to show that it was recessively inherited. He postulated that this was caused by a mutation in a gene encoding an enzyme involved in the metabolism of a class of compounds called alkaptons. He was then the first to propose the idea that some diseases were *"inborn errors of metabolism"* and that *"one gene produces one protein"*. This is the molecular basis of inheritance and signalled the birth of clinical genetics.

It was almost 40 years later, using mouldy bread, that Garrod's hypothesis of 'one gene one protein' would finally be experimentally proved. In 1941 George Beadle and Edward Tatum saw that exposing moulds to radiation reduced their growth as a result of inhibiting their ability to produce essential nutrients. However, providing the mutated mould with a specific supplement allowed the mould to continue growing again. It was therefore concluded that each mutation must inactivate the enzyme (protein) needed to synthesize the nutrient. For this, they won the Nobel prize in 1958.

One day, in 1911, the American Thomas Hunt Morgan, whilst working on his fruit-fly experiments, noticed a single male fly in one of his culture bottles that had white-eyes, instead of red. Out of curiosity, he bred the fly with a normal red-eyed female. This produced offspring that all had red-eyes. Crossing these offspring produced an F2 generation with some white-eyed flies, similar to Mendel's peas, except all these white-eyed flies were male. From this he postulated that the X-chromosome carries discrete hereditary units he described as genes; a term recently introduced by Wilhelm Johannsen in 1909. He further found other genetic variations that were also sex-linked and usually inherited together leading him to conclude that genes were arranged in linear fashion on chromosomes. In 1933 he was awarded the Nobel prize that was followed by further Nobel prizes for a number of his students including George Beadle and Hermann Joseph Muller.

Interestingly, his great-grandfather, Francis Scott Key, wrote the *Star-Spangled Banner.*

Frederick Griffith was employed by the British government during World War II to develop a vaccine against Spanish flu. During his experiments, he discovered that a harmless strain of *Streptococcus pneumoniae* could be made lethal again after being exposed to a heat-killed virulent strain. This lethal virulent bacterium strain had a polysaccharide capsule giving it a smooth surface appearance in contrast to the harmless strain with a rough surface due to a lack of the capsule. When the dead virulent strain bacteria, killed by heating and so not lethal to mice, were mixed with live harmless strain bacteria they become lethal. Amazingly, the live bacteria from the dead mice all had smooth surfaces; this meant that the harmless rough surface bacteria had acquired the ability to make capsules from the dead smooth-surfaced bacteria. He hypothesised that a "transforming principle" was passed between the bacteria. However, before he could go further to identify

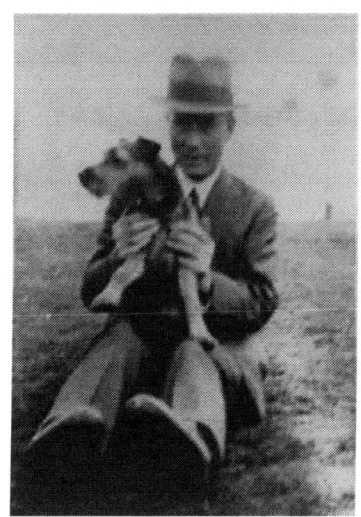

Frederick Griffith

this component, he was killed during the London Blitz in 1941. His death hardly received any mention.

Three scientists, Oswald Avery, Colin MacLeod, and Maclyn McCarty, then followed up the work shortly after Frederick Griffith's death to determined what the mysterious "transforming principle" – a substance that could cause a heritable change of bacterial cells - was. Repeating his experiments, they purified DNA, proteins and other materials separately from the virulent smooth *Streptococcus pneumoniae* strain that they mixed with the harmless rough-surfaced bacteria. Only those mixed with DNA were "transformed" into virulent bacteria and acquired the smooth capsule. This amazing discovery, in many ways, radically changed the direction of genetics driving research towards the study of DNA structure and sequences. Incredibly, this work was neglected by the Nobel Foundation, which did later express regret for the omission.

Earlier in the 1920s, Phoebus Levene, a Russian who had emigrated to the U.S to avoid anti-Semitism, identified the components of DNA as a purine or pyrimidine base, a pentose sugar and a phosphate group base that were linked together to form phosphate-sugar-base units and that DNA consisted of a string of these linked together. Another emigrant to the U.S., this time fleeing anti-Semitism in Nazi Germany, Erwin Chargaff demonstrated that DNA showed a pattern where the number of guanine bases equalled the number of cytosines and the number of adenines was the same as the number of thymines in any DNA sample. He mentioned some of his newest results to Crick and Watson a year before they published their model of DNA structure.

Using X-ray crystallography - a technique for determining a molecule's three-dimensional structure by analysing the X-ray diffraction patterns of crystals made up of the molecule in question - to study DNA, Rosalind Franklin and her student Raymond Gosling, at King's College in London produced a very famous image of DNA. This allowed her to see that the sugar-phosphate backbone of DNA lies on the outside of the molecule (not the inside as was previously thought) and that DNA has a helical structure of two DNA strands (not three as proposed in competing theories). She was also able to determine the

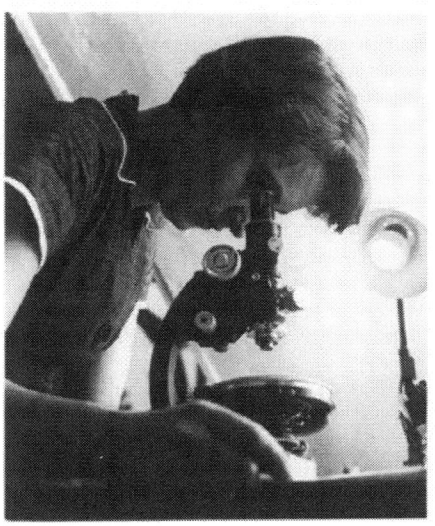

Rosalind Franklin

size of the double helix. Her boss at King's College presented Franklin's data and unpublished conclusions to Watson and Crick, supposedly without her knowledge.

Francis Crick and James Watson already knew DNA contained equal ratios of C and G residues and A and T residues, thanks to Chargaff, and now they knew from Rosalind Franklin's X-ray data that DNA must consist of two anti-parallel chains, the backbone had to be on the outside, and they knew the size of the helix. Cutting out cardboard templates of the four DNA bases and playing with them on their cramped desk at Cambridge University, they found that lining up an A-T pair showed an identical in shape to a G-C pair. These could, therefore, be the equal steps of DNA's spiral staircase; each of the four letters on one chain is matched by its opposite on the other; when the chains separate, each is the template for a new chain of exactly matching sequence, allowing DNA to replicate. Putting all these pieces of the puzzle together, they published their model for the structure of DNA alongside Franklin's own report, and together with Wilkins they went on to win the Nobel Prize in 1962. By this time, Rosalind had died of ovarian cancer four years earlier, aged 37.

Though many of the pieces were now known, it was still not clear how everything fitted together. Now the riddle was, how the four bases of DNA can provide instructions for the twenty different amino acids that form proteins, and how the related RNA fitted in? This promoted James Watson and George Gamow in 1954 to form the RNA Tie Club, a scientific gentleman's club of select members who could share their ideas and latest findings. Meeting twice a year the 20, all male, members representing each amino acid, with an additional four honorary members representing each nucleotide, all received woollen ties with an embroidered helix on them. Though meetings generally involved many cigars and much alcohol they did indeed develop and foster many influential ideas and concepts and eight of these members went on to win Nobel Prizes.

Russian-born, Gamow was a highly gifted theoretical physicist being elected a member of the Academy of Sciences of the USSR at age 28, one of the youngest ever — after a number of major discoveries. However, increasing oppression pushed him and his wife to flee Russia. He once paddled a kayak for 36 hours over the Black Sea and on another occasion attempted to paddle through the ice-cold Barents Sea to Norway; poor weather foiled both attempts. However, a year later, in 1933, they both managed to obtain permission to attend a physics conference in Brussels, where they promptly defected and moved to the US. There he lectured in physics and researched the Big Bang theory. It was only in his later years that Gamow started working in biology and applying his amazing reasoning and creativity. It was in this environment of collaboration that Gamow postulated that a nucleotide code consisting of three letters would be enough to define all 20 amino acids, i.e. the concept of the "codon". Sydney Brenner then provided experimental evidence for the codon and Francis Crick proposed the *"Adaptor hypothesis"* that molecules (later discovered and called transfer RNAs) ferried the amino acids around, and put them in the correct order corresponding to the nucleic acid sequence.

However, it was a non-member of the RNA tie club, Marshall Nirenberg, who together with his team of co-workers, cracked the DNA and RNA code. His brilliant idea was to produce RNA consisting only of one base – uracil (a nucleotide specific only to RNA

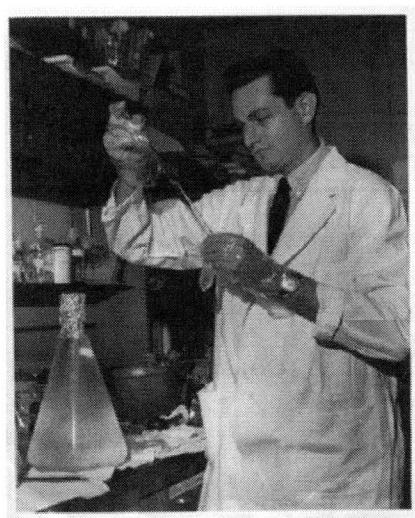

Marshall Nirenberg

and equivalent to the T in DNA). They added this to a mixture containing the cellular machinery for protein synthesis, extracted from *E.coli*. They then added the 20 amino acids, but being sure to radio-label only one of them. They consequently found that in the extract containing the radioactively labelled phenylalanine, the resulting protein was also radioactive leading them to conclude that they had found the genetic code for phenylalanine: UUU (three uracil bases in a row) on RNA. Within a few years, his research team had performed similar experiments and found that three-base repeats of adenosine (AAA) produced the amino acid lysine, and cytosine repeats (CCC) produced proline. Nirenberg was awarded the Nobel prize in 1968, for these discoveries and his work led to the race to discover the whole genetic code for all 64 codons and their respective 20 amino acids which was completed over the following six years.

Next, the search for the location and sequences of different genes began. Before the completion of the human genome project, many expected our genome to contain in the region of 100,000 genes based on the assumption that because we are one of the most complex creatures on Earth, we should have more genes. However, it appears we only have

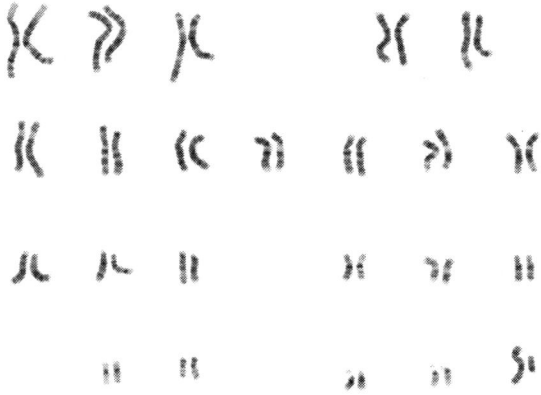

A human karyogram stained using Giemsa dye (G-banding)

around 20,000-25,000 genes; a similar number to a chimpanzee or a mouse. It is obviously crucial to be able to identify genes and their sequences if they are to be researched and used for diagnostics. Mapping of the human genome began over 100 years ago when in 1911, the gene responsible for red-green colour blindness, was assigned to the X chromosome following the observation that this disorder was passed on in an X-linked inheritance pattern to sons by unaffected mothers. Subsequently, many other disorders affecting only males were likewise mapped to the X chromosome. In the 1970s came the discovery of a staining technique called G-banding, from the Giemsa dye, which made the identification of each chromosome much easier with characteristic darker and lighter bands serving as rough landmarks on the chromosomes. This led to the assignment of around 1,000 genes to specific chromosomes such as the gene leading to Tay Sachs disease found on a particular area of chromosome 15.

A further development of this technique relied on known variable sequences in the genome as markers for nearby abnormal genes. This was first developed by Kan and Dozy, in 1978, who noted that near the sickle cell gene was a stretch of DNA which varied (i.e. polymorphic) between most Africans and African-Americans and which could be used as a marker in a given family for linkage with the sickle cell gene. Using polymorphic sequences of DNA with no known function to serve as markers in linking with the inheritance of a disease in a family allowed scientists to analyse very large families to determine which individuals inherited a disease in combination with one of the many different markers on

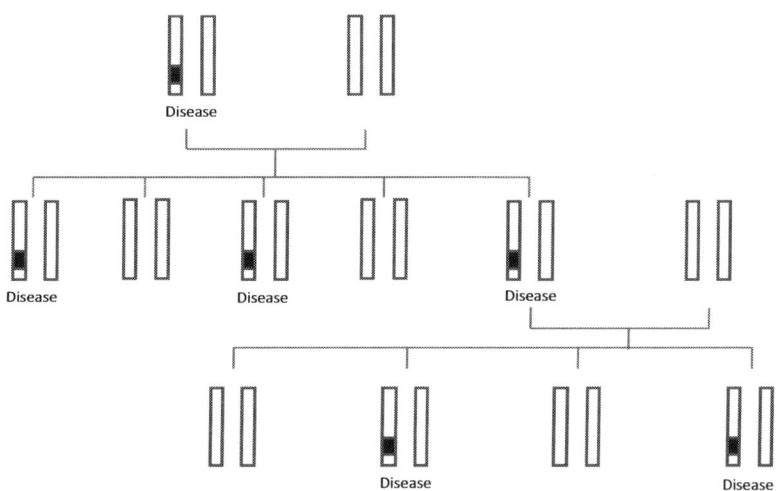

Finding a chromosome marker (black) linked to development of a
dominantly inherited disease

283

different chromosomes. This led to an explosion in the knowledge of genes' chromosomal whereabouts with around 2,000 genes being mapped by 1991. For example, this included pinpointing the location of the Huntington's disease gene to Chromosome 4 using families in Venezuela and the gene for cystic fibrosis on Chromosome 7.

In 1977 Frederick Sanger, at Cambridge University, developed a method to sequence the DNA of genes. He received his second Nobel prize for this. The method used dideoxynucleotides, a type of nucleotide that when bound to a growing DNA sequence, terminates replication as they cannot bind other bases. A sequencing reaction is performed using four reactions each containing a small quantity of one of the A-, T-, G-, or C-dideoxynucleotides together in nucleotide mix of all four bases. Different lengths of growing sequences will finish ending in an A, T G or C the end depending on when a dideoxynucleotide is added in each of the reactions. By running the samples from the four reactions on a gel that separates the DNA lengths you can piece together the sequence.

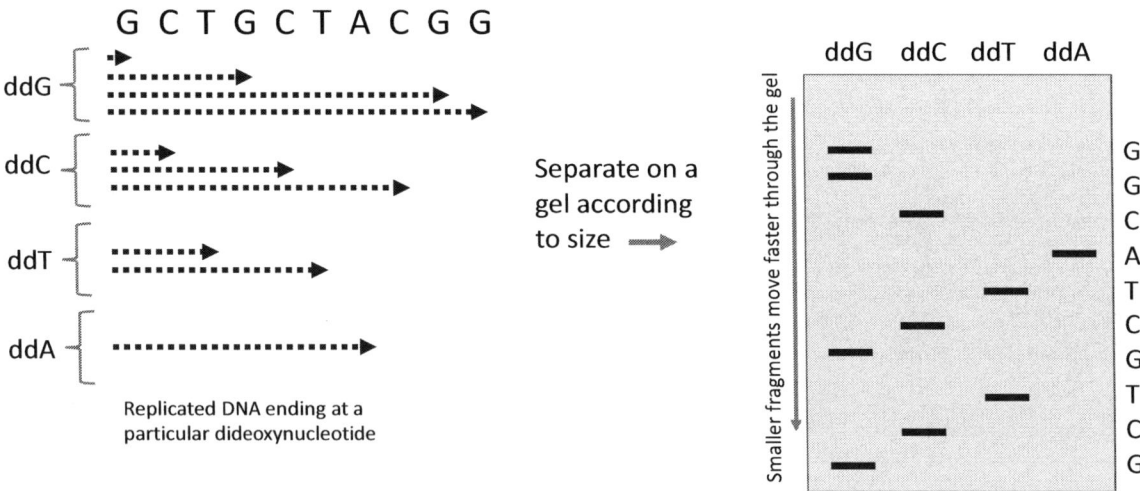

Sanger DNA sequencing: C, G, T and A dideoxynucleotide reactions are performed that result in different lengths of DNA ending in A C, G, T or a that are separated by size using a gel

284

However, to perform molecular experiments with DNA including large-scale sequencing, relatively large quantities of DNA were needed. In 1983, Kary Mullis devised and developed a breakthrough method to enable the amplification of DNA, using the polymerase chain reaction, known as PCR. PCR consists of repeated cycles of elevated temperatures to separate DNA strands, which are then copied by a heat-stable DNA polymerase, extracted from a strain of bacteria that live in hot springs, first found in Yellowstone Park. Repeating the cycle many times leads to an exponential increase in the quantity of DNA. He was working for a biotech firm at the time and thought it was a *"long-shot experiment"* and described leaving the lab at midnight after pouring himself a cold Becks into a pre-chilled 500ml beaker from the isotope freezer for luck before returning next

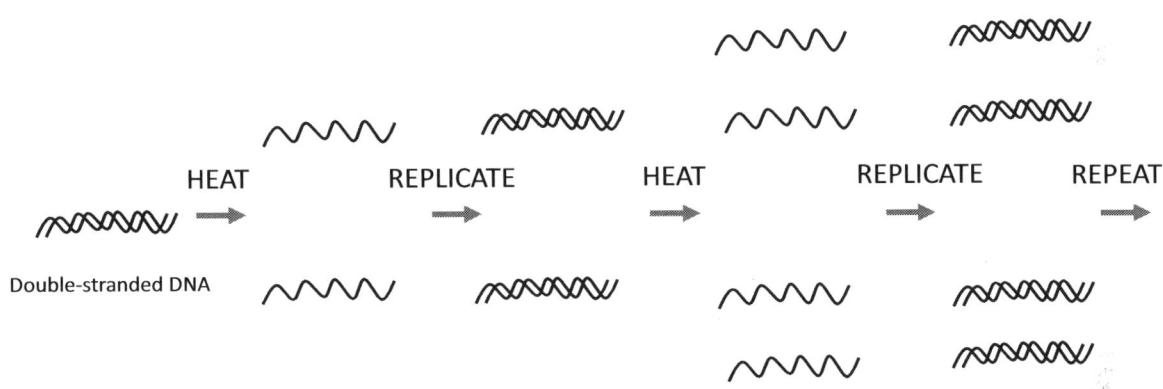

PCR: double stranded DNA is heated to make single-stranded. This is replicated using DNA polymerase and heated to separate again. This cycle is repeated for up to 30 times or more

morning for the results. Incredibly, his findings were initially rejected from several well-known scientific journals, before being published in the lesser-known journal *Methods in Enzymology*, for which he received the Nobel Prize in Chemistry in 1993. This method revolutionised molecular biology and genetics. Using this method, even traces of DNA can

285

be amplified into amounts that can be easily sequenced or quantified. A controversial figure, he often suggested that he thought up the idea whilst on drugs; *"What if I had not taken LSD ever; would I have still invented PCR? I don't know. I doubt it. I seriously doubt it."* Following his Nobel prize, he became an avid surfer and, in his biography, described an alien encounter in the form of a racoon. He died in 2019 aged 74-years-old. I have poster of him and his surfboard on my office wall.

In 1990 the Human Genome Project was started to sequence the entire human genome based on the use of the Sanger sequencing technology together with PCR. Sequencing machines soon improved based on Sanger's method with machines running 96 sequences at a time, at 500,000 bases per day. This form of sequencing became the main tool for the completion of the human genome project and in 2003 a draft version of the sequences of the 3 billion chemical base pairs making up human DNA was published.

Since then, the development of new techniques in sequencing, known as next-generation sequencing, can enable the human genome to be sequenced very rapidly, compared to the many years with the Sanger methods. These new methods uses array-based sequencing which combine the techniques developed in Sanger sequencing to process millions of reactions in parallel, at very high speed and throughput with a reduced cost. A full human genome can now be sequenced within an hours for only a few hundred pounds. This has enabled the UK, for example, to start and finish the 100,000 human genome project. It may well be that everyone in the future have their genomes sequenced as part of routine healthcare.

In the 1980s, methods became available to allow easy ways to produce proteins, such as the insulin protein, deficient in diabetics, or clotting factors missing in patients with haemophilia. This is done by introducing human genes into bacterial DNA so that the modified bacteria can then produce the corresponding protein, known as a recombinant protein, which can be harvested from the bacteria and injected in people who cannot produce it naturally. Millions of diabetics worldwide use recombinant insulin, made in both bacteria and yeast, to regulate their blood sugar levels.

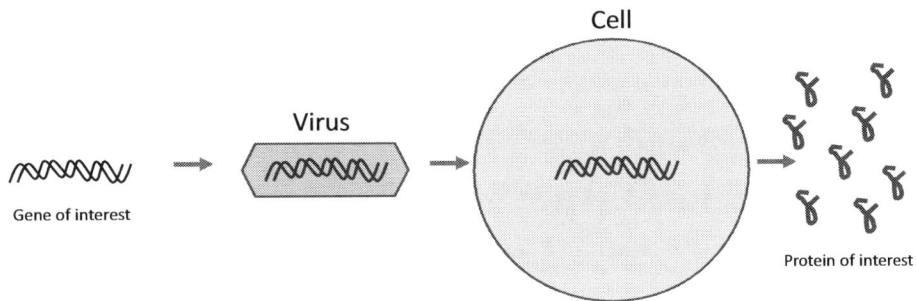

DNA containing a gene can be inserted into a cell, using a virus, that the cell uses to make protein

Scientists took the next step of introducing genes straight into human cells, focusing on diseases caused by single-gene defects, such as cystic fibrosis, haemophilia, muscular dystrophy and sickle cell anaemia. The idea is that cells such as the patient's liver or lung cells are infected with a modified virus, used to carry a therapeutic human gene, into a cell previously lacking that gene enabling it to produce a functional protein. The generation of a functional protein product from the therapeutic gene restores the target cell to a normal state. On September 14th 1990, the first approved gene therapy trial was launched. A 4-year-old girl named Ashanthi DeSilva underwent treatment for the rare genetic disease, severe combined immunodeficiency. DeSilva lacked a key enzyme called adenosine deaminase, which left her immune system crippled and put her at constant risk of contracting an infection that could kill her. A viral vector was used to introduce a functional copy of the adenosine deaminase gene into her white blood cells, improving her immune

287

system function and allowing her to live a normal life for the first time, without having to be isolated to avoid infection. However, this procedure was not a cure; the cells treated genetically only work for a few months, so the process had to be repeated every few months. Though authorities were originally supportive of the development of this gene therapy work, all changed in 1999 when a patient died as a result of gene therapy. Jesse Gelsinger, an 18-year-old born without a gene for ornithine trancarbamylase, suffered a massive immune response following gene therapy.

Many gene therapy trials were stopped as a result and there was a focus towards developing safer gene therapies with newer viruses. China became the first nation to approve a gene therapy for head and neck cancer in 2003, followed by Russia's approval of a therapy for peripheral artery disease in 2011. In 2012 the EU approved a therapy for treating lipoprotein lipase deficiency. Half a dozen other gene therapies have since been approved in the EU such as for beta-thalassemia. The US has experienced a similar boom, and it is thought that by 2030 we could see over fifty cell and gene therapy launches. Currently, as of 2019, nearly 2,600 gene therapy clinical trials have been completed, are ongoing or have been approved worldwide in a variety of diseases including haemophilia, Fabry disease, Huntington's disease, sickle cell disease, and various types of cancers. It is estimated that around 500,000 patients will have been treated with gene therapy products by 2030.

In 2018, a Chinese scientist announced that he had created the world's first genome-edited babies. The twin girls reportedly had their DNA for a gene called CCR5 deleted whilst they were embryos, following IVF, to make them immune to infection by HIV, the virus that causes AIDS and needs the CCR5 protein to infect cells. This used a newly developed gene-editing technology, called CRISPR. This involves using a piece of

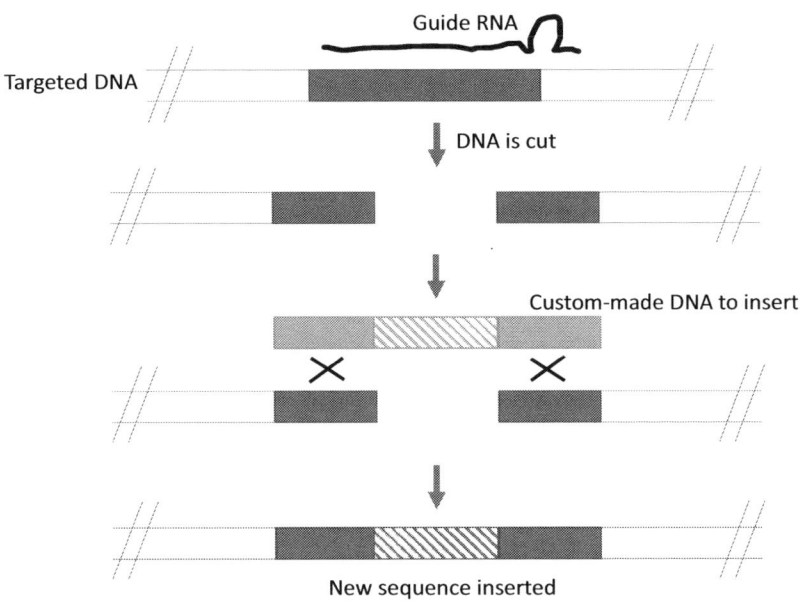

CRISPR: a specific guide RNA pinpoints to cut a section of DNA
and allows the insertion of a new piece of DNA.

bacterial DNA that behaves like a sat-nav, homing in on a specific location in a genome where a cutting enzyme snips out the bit of DNA which is replaced by a new sequence of choice. Genome editing may have great potential for dealing with inherited genetic disorders. For example, one therapy involves taking a patient's own cells, editing them outside the body to produce high levels of haemoglobin, then reintroducing the engineered cells back into the body as a treatment for beta-thalassaemia. Such a therapeutic approach for the treatment of inherited eye diseases is also thought to offer good prospects.

Returning to the Chinese experiment it is important to remember that any changes made in human embryos could be passed down for generations, which is why this sort of genetic manipulation has long been considered unethical as it is possible to change the entire human gene pool. Indeed the whole "experiment" received widespread criticism.

In the future genetics will continue to have an important impact on society. In the future, medicine will be tailored to a person's genetic sequences or genome, and their environmental history and lifestyle. Rather than a one-size-fits-most treatment, doctors will use genetic data to determine what therapies one should receive based on genetic traits they have inherited. Perhaps people may become discriminated against and judged simply on their genetic sequences. Perhaps it may become more common-place to have our DNA sequences artificially modified. However, understanding and appreciating one's genetic sequences will allow people to be able to take more control of their health to choose lifestyles that reduce the risks of disease, understand their environmental risks, and inform tailor-made treatments.

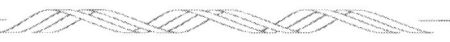

# Glossary

Allele: One of alternative forms of a genetic sequence.

Amino Acid: The building blocks of proteins.

Autosome: A chromosome which is not a sex chromosome.

Base pair (bp): The fundamental unit of a double stranded DNA molecule, (more strictly - a nucleotide pair). The base Adenine on one strand is paired with Thymine on the other and Guanine with Cytosine. The lengths of double stranded DNA molecules are frequently given in bp (or nucleotide pairs).

Chromosome: The structure which is built up around each nuclear DNA molecule.

Codon: A sequence of three adjacent DNA or RNA nucleotides that codes for a specific amino acid in the synthesis of a protein molecule.

Congenital: Present at birth but not necessarily inherited.

Consanguineous mating: A mating in which male and female are related by descent, i.e. inbreeding.

Deletion: A mutation resulting in the loss of normal DNA sequence. A deletion may be of any size from 1 nucleotide pair to the loss of a piece of chromosome.

DNA: The molecule in which the genetic information of most organisms is encoded.

Dominant: An allele is dominant if its effect can be observed in the phenotype of a heterozygote.

Eukaryote: A class of organisms in which the genetic material is contained within a nucleus.

Enzyme: Proteins that speeds up the rate of a chemical reaction in a living organism.

Founder effect: A high frequency of a particular allele in a population caused by it having been present in one or more members of a small number of individuals from whom the population is descended.

Gene: A region of DNA which contains the information to create either a polypeptide chain, known as a protein, or a functional RNA.

Genetic Drift: Random changes in allele frequencies from one generation to another in small populations

Genotype: The alleles present in an individual at the locus under consideration.

Germline: cells which develop into eggs and sperm or inherited material that comes from the eggs or sperm and is passed on to offspring.

Heterozygote: An individual having two different alleles at a locus.

Heterozygous advantage: A situation where heterozygous genotypes are more fit than homozygous genotypes.

Hormone: A chemical substance produced in the body that controls and regulates the activity of certain cells or organs.

Karyotype: The chromosomal constitution of an individual.

Nucleotide: A building block of a nucleic acid consisting of a base (adenine, thymine, cytosine, guanine, uracil) joined to a sugar (ribose or deoxyribose) and a phosphate.

Phenotype: An individual's outward appearance.

Polymorphism: Genetic variation occurring in a population so that at least two alleles are present at a frequency of 1 percent or greater.

Prokaryote: A simpler organism than a eukaryote having no nucleus. e.g. a bacterium.

Recessive: A mutation or allele which does not affect the phenotype unless it is homozygous.

RNA: The class of molecules which are the primary products of genes.

Sex Chromosome: One of the chromosomes which are present in different numbers in males and females. In humans this means the X and Y chromosomes, XX in females and XY in males.

Syndrome: A collection of symptoms which occur together and are thought to be caused by the same mutation or chromosomal anomaly.

Transcription: The process of copying DNA into RNA.

X (or sex) linked: A gene which is present on the X chromosome.

# Further Reading

**WHAT IS CELL, DNA, MUTATION, PROTEIN, CHROMOSOME?**

Molecular Biology of the Cell. Bruce Alberts.

**GENETIC INHERITANCE**

Lewin's genes XII. Jocelyn E. Krebs, Elliott S. Goldstein, Stephen T. Kilpatrick.

On the Origin of Mendelian Genetics. Sandler I, Sandler L. American Zoologist 1986 26, 3: 753-768.

A medical history of the Spanish Habsburgs. As traced in portraits. Hodge GP. JAMA. 1977 Sep 12;238(11):1169-74.

Familiarity breeds: incest and the Ptolemaic Dynasty. Ager SL. J Hell Stud. 2005;125:1-34.

Pycnodysostosis: the disease of Henri de Toulouse-Lautrec. Markatos K, Mavrogenis AF, Karamanou M, Androutsos G. Eur J Orthop Surg Traumatol. 2018. 28:1569-1572.

Haemophilia in the Descendants of Queen Victoria. English Monarchs. Accessed July 2 2019.

Mystery Solved: The Identification of the Two Missing Romanov Children Using DNA Analysis. Coble MD, Loreille OM, Wadhams MJ, Edson SM, Maynard K, Meyer CE, Niederstätter H, Berger C, Berger B, Falsetti AB, Gill P, Parson W, Finelli LN. PLoS One. 2009; 4(3): e4838.

Genomic analysis of family data reveals additional genetic effects on intelligence and personality. Hill WD, Arslan RC, Xia C, Luciano M, Amador C, Navarro P, Hayward C, Nagy R, Porteous DJ, McIntosh AM, Deary IJ, Haley CS, Penke L. Mol Psychiatry. 2018. 23: 2347-2362.

Searching for neurological diseases in the Julio-Claudian dynasty of the Roman Empire. Camargo CHF, Teive HAG. Arq Neuropsiquiatr. 2018. 76: 53-57.

Facts About Angelman Syndrome 7th Edition. Williams CA, Peters SU, Calculator, SN. Angelman Syndrome Foundation. Jan 1, 2009.

On Island of the Colorblind, Paradise Has a Different Hue. Sone D. National Geographic. Jan 26 2018.

## CHROMOSOMAL DISORDERS

Essential Medical Genetics: Edward S. Tobias, Michael Connor, Malcolm Ferguson–Smith.

Eddie the male tortoiseshell kitten who is Britain's rarest cat. The Daily Mail. Aug 26 2009.

Intersex and the Olympic Games. Ritchie R, Reynard J, Lewis T. J R Soc Med. 2008. 101: 395–399.

A terrible crime with two victims. Manchester Evening News. Aug 13 2010.

Genes, Brain Function, and Behavior: What Genes Do, How They Malfunction, and Ways to Repair Damage. Wahlsten D. Academic Press, Mar 14 2019.

Trans History. deCarlo T. Lulu.com. 2018.

Tula: I am a woman: Interview with Caroline Cossey. Margaux S, Dallas D. International TransScript. 1992. 2, 2, 18-22.

## SKELETAL DISORDERS

Hall JG, Flora C, Scott C, Pauli RM, Tanak K. (2004) "Majewski Osteodysplastic Primordial Dwarfism Type II (MOPD II): Natural History and Clinical Findings American Journal of Medical Genetics 130A:55-72

"Secret History" The Strangest Viking (TV Episode 2003)

Pycnodysostosis and the making of an artist. Hodder A, Huntley C, Aronson JK, Ramachandran M. Gene. 2015 Jan 15;555(1):59-62.

Pseudoachondroplasia and the seven Ovitz siblings who survived Auschwitz. Muensterer OJ1, Berdon WE, Lachman RS, Done SL. Pediatr Radiol. 2012 Apr;42(4):475-80. doi: 10.1007/s00247-012-2364-8. Epub 2012 Mar 18.

Ellis-van Creveld syndrome: its history. Muensterer OJ, Berdon W, McManus C, Oestreich A, Lachman RS, Cohen MM Jr, Done S. Pediatr Radiol. 2013 Aug;43(8):1030-6.

Egill Skallagrímsson: the first case of Van Buchem disease? Stride P. J R Coll Physicians Edinb. 2011 Jun;41(2):169-73.

The skeleton in the closet. Kaplan FS. Gene. 2013 Oct 1;528(1):7-11.

Abraham Lincoln's marfanoid mother: the earliest known case of multiple endocrine neoplasia type 2B? Sotos JG. Clin Dysmorphol. 2012 Jul;21(3):131-6.

Illness and art: the legacy of Paul Klee. Varga J. Curr Opin Rheumatol. 2004 Nov;16(6):714-7.

## CONNECTIVE TISSUE DISORDERS

Rachmaninov and Marfan's syndrome. Young DA. Br Med J (Clin Res Ed). 1986 Dec 20-27;293(6562):1624-6.

Creativity and chronic disease. Niccolo Paganini (1782-1840). Wolf P. West J Med. 2001 Nov;175(5):345.

20-year-old with condition which makes her age dramatically undergoes facelift. Gladwell. The Metro. Feb 16 2017

## MUSCULAR DISORDERS

Myotonic dystrophy in Ancient Egypt. Cattaino G, Vicario L Eur Neurol. 1999;41(2):59-63.

Of sad and wished-for years: Elizabeth Barrett Browning's lifelong illness. Buchanan A1, Weiss EB. Perspect Biol Med. 2011 Autumn;54(4):479-503.

Gross muscle hypertrophy in whippet dogs is caused by a mutation in the myostatin gene. Shelton GD, Engvall E. Neuromuscul Disord. 2007 Oct; 1:721-2.

## DERMATOLOGICAL DISORDERS

Skin Disease. 4th Edition. Habif T, Dinulos J. Chapman S, Zug K.

The face is familiar... Michael Berryman. Monahan M. The Telegraph. 17 Mar 2006.

Early history of the different forms of neurofibromatosis from ancient Egypt to the British Empire and beyond: First descriptions, medical curiosities, misconceptions, landmarks, and the persons behind the syndromes. Ruggieri M, Praticò AD, Caltabiano R, Polizzi A. Am J Med Genet A. 2018; 176(3):515-550.

Clinical and historical aspects of the Elephant Man: exploring the facts and the myths. Huntley C, Hodder A, Ramachandran M. Gene. 2015 Jan 15;555(1):63-5.

## HAIR DISORDERS

Alopecia areata: A review. Amin SS, Sachdeva S. Journal of the Saudi Society of Dermatology & Dermatologic Surgery. 2013 17, 2, 37-45.

Victorian spectacle: Julia Pastrana, the bearded and hairy female. Browne J, Messenger S. Endeavour. 2003 Dec;27(4):155-9.

Merry Wiesner-Hanks, The Marvelous Hairy Girls: The Gonzales Sisters and Their Worlds ( New Haven: Yale University Press, 2009)

## RESPIRATORY DISORDERS

Physiological basis of cystic fibrosis: a historical perspective. Quinton PM. Physiol Rev. 1999 Jan;79(1 Suppl):S3-S22.

Cystic fibrosis--a probable cause of Frédéric Chopin's suffering and death. Majka L1, Goździk J, Witt M. J Appl Genet. 2003;44(1):77-84.

An overview of alpha-1 antitrypsin deficiency. Hericks AJ1, Bhat A. Mo Med. 2007 May-Jun;104(3):255-9.

## HEART DISORDERS

Inherited heart conditions. NHS https://www.nhsinform.scot/illnesses-and-conditions/heart-and-blood-vessels/conditions/inherited-heart-conditions

Noonan's Syndrome: A Historical Perspective. Cole RB. Pediatrics. 1980, 66, 3.

Genetic disorders in portraits. Emery AE. Am J Med Genet. 1996 Dec 18;66(3):334-9.

Genetics of Human Cardiovascular Disease. Kathiresan S, Srivastava D. Cell. 2012 Mar 16; 148(6): 1242–1257.

Cardiac Ion Channelopathies and the Sudden Infant Death Syndrome. Wilders R. ISRN Cardiol. 2012; 2012: 846171.

## LIVER DISORDERS

Genetics in liver diseases: From diagnostics to precise therapy. Weber SN, Lammert F. Clin Liver Dis (Hoboken). 2017. 9: 1-4.

Former Olympian, pro football player Howard Dell competes in Transplant Games. Olsen C. Michigan Live. Jul 30, 2012

Student refused entry to clubs because her slurred speech and staggering made her look 'drunk' is told deadly illness is causing her symptoms. Pickles K. The Daily Mail. Jan 26 2016.

The Ongoing Mystery Of Hemingway's Misdiagnosed Death: Accident, Suicide Or Genetic Disorder? Olson S. Medical Daily. Jul 2, 2013

The Real Code of Leonardo da Vinci. Ose L. Curr Cardiol Rev. 2008 Feb; 4(1): 60–62.

The surreal thing: the return of Noel Fielding. Armstrong S. Evening Standard. 31 July 2014

## KIDNEY DISORDERS

Alport Syndrome. Watson S, Bush JS.StatPearls [Internet]. Treasure Island (FL): StatPearls Publishing; 2019-2018 Dec 15.

Maestro, Marguerite, morphine: The last years in the life of Mikhail Bulgakov.

Zilberstein G, Maor U, Baskin E, Righetti PG. J Proteomics. 2016 Jan 10;131:199-204.

What was wrong with Tiny Tim? Lewis DW. Am J Dis Child. 1992. 146: 1403-7.

Polycystic kidney disease: antiquity to the 20th century. Torres VE,Watson ML. Nephrol Dial Transplant (1998) 13: 2690–2696

## DIGESTIVE DISORDERS

Alfred the Great: a diagnosis. Craig, G Journal of the Royal Society of Medicine. 1991. 84 (5): 303–05.

Joe C. Dead at Twenty-Six. Dansby A. November 17, 2000.

Ex-Street star thanks nurses after baby fight. Manchester Evening News. 2004, 9 Aug.

Crohn's disease. Baumgart DC, Sandborn WJ Lancet. 2012 380 (9853): 1590–605.

Coeliac disease. Di Sabatino A Corazza GR. Lancet. 2009; 373: 1480-1493

## BLOOD DISORDERS

Walter Clement Noel—first patient described with sickle cell disease. Steensma DP, Kyle RA, Shampo MA. Mayo Clin Proc. 2010 Oct;85(10):e74-5.

Hicks, Tameka L. (2008). "T-Boz: Fighting against the odds". USA Weekend. Archived from the original on November 4, 2013.

TLC's Tionne 'T-Boz' Watkins on living with sickle cell disease.ABC NEWS. Sep 12, 2017.

Sickle Cell and the Social Sciences: Health, Racism and Disablement. Dyson SM. Routledge. 2019.

Pechstein zitiert E-Mail und beantragt Startrecht, Spiegel Online (in German), 15 February

2010

Hereditary spherocytosis. Perrotta S, Gallagher PG, Mohandas. Lancet. 2008. 372 (9647): 1411–26.

The Thalassemias: Disorders of Globin Synthesis. Weatherall DJ. Williams Hematology (9e ed.). McGraw Hill Professional. 2015

Clay soils Pete's record. 23 May, 2002 http://news.bbc.co.uk/sport2/hi/tennis/french_open/1952120.stm.

Glucose-6-phosphate dehydrogenase deficiency: a historical perspective. Beutler E. Blood 2008 111:16-24;

Vincent van Gogh: a pathographic analysis. Correa R. Med Hypotheses. 2014 Feb;82(2):141-4.

Born to the Purple: the Story of Porphyria. Lane N. Scientific American. on December 16, 2002.

The Real-life diseases that spread the vampire myth. Dowling S. 2016. http://www.bbc.com/future/story/20161031-the-real-life-disease-that-spread-the-vampire-myth

Truncated erythropoietin receptor causes dominantly inherited benign human erythrocytosis. de la Chapelle. A; Traskelin AL; Juvonen E. PNAS. 1993. 90 (10): 4495–9.

Fanconi anaemia and cancer: an intricate relationship. Nalepa G, Clapp DW. Nat Rev Cancer. 2018 Mar;18(3):168-185.

Little Frankenstein,' conceived so Minnesota doctors could save sister, is now a happy teen. Olson J. Star Tribune JUNE 25, 2017

Genotype analysis identifies the cause of the "royal disease". Rogaev EI, Grigorenko AP, Faskhutdinova G, Kittler EL, Moliaka YK. Science. 2009 6;326:817.

Past, present and future of hemophilia: a narrative review. Franchini M, Mannucci PM. Orphanet J Rare Dis. 2012; 7: 24.

von Willebrand Disease: A Concise Review and Update for the Practicing Physician. Swami A, Kaur V. Clin Appl Thromb Hemost. 2017. 23(8):900-910.

New Insights Into the Treatment of Glanzmann Thrombasthenia. Poon MC, Di Minno G, d'Oiron R, Zotz R. Transfusion Medicine Reviews. 2016. 30, 2: 92-99.

Doctors link skater's death to genetic defect. Pincus A CNN News. June 28, 1996.

## IMMUNE DISORDERS

Edward Jenner and the history of smallpox and vaccination. Riedel S. Proc (Bayl Univ Med Cent). 2005 Jan; 18(1): 21–25.

'Boy in the Bubble' Moved a World He Couldn't Touch. C Haberman. The New York Times. Dec. 9, 2015

"Severe combined immunodeficiencies: New and Old Scenarios". Aloj G, Giardano G, Valentino L, Maio F, Gallo V, Esposito T, Naddei R, Cirillo E, Pignata C. Int Rev Immunol. (2012). 31 (1): 43–65.

Autoimmunity: From Bench to Bedside. Anaya JM, Shoenfeld Y, Rojas-Villarraga A, et al. Bogota (Colombia): El Rosario University Press; 2013.

Bush Water Supply Studied for Link to Graves' Disease : Health: The Secret Service is checking four present or former homes for unusual levels of iodine and lithium. Cimons M. Los Angles Times. May 29, 1991

Lenin: A Biography. Service R. McMillan Publishers. 2000.

"Marty Feldman: "Damn your eyes!"". Amc.com. Retrieved 5 Jan 2019.

Good, bad 'days'. Factor S,. Los Angeles Times. JULY 12, 1987

Historical Descriptions of Multiple Sclerosis. Pearce J.M.S. Eur Neurol 2005;54:49–53

Comedian Richard Pryor dies at 65. CNN News. Dec 11, 2005

The History of Lupus Erythematosus and Discoid Lupus: From Hippocrates to the Present. Norman A. Lupus Open Access 2016, 1:1

Seal opens up about Lupus battle as he teams up with Myleene Klass and Nile Rodgers for NHS charity single. Evans M. Metro.co.uk July 5 2018.

Living with lupus, Elaine Paige. Burne J. The Times. June 7 2004

Lady Gaga's 'borderline positive' comment sheds light on lupus. Park M. CNN June 3, 2010

Fibromyalgia: the chronic pain that thwarted Lady Gaga's tour. Robinson A. The Guardian. 19 Sep 2017.

Toni Braxton Released From Hospital After Lupus Flare-Up. Kreps D. The Rolling Stone. OCT4, 2016.

Selena Gomez undergoes kidney transplant following battle with lupus. Mairs P. The

Independent. Sep 14 2017.

## ENDOCRINE DISORDERS

The Endocrine System, 2nd Editio. Raven JH, Raven P, Chew S. Churchill Livingstone. 2010

Franz Josef Kallmann (1897–1965) -- Pioneer in Neurology. Stahnisch FW, Pow S. Journal of Neurology 2016. 266:1-3

Jimmy Scott obituary. Williams R. The Guardian. Jun 15 2014.

X-linked nephrogenic diabetes insipidus mutations in North America and the Hopewell hypothesis. Bichet DG, Rosenthal W, Didwania A. J Clin Invest. 1993. 92:1262-1268.

How an Irish giant and an 18th-century surgeon could help people with growth disorders. Parry V. The Guardian. Jan 11 2011

Hereditary Gigantism-the biblical giant Goliath and his brothers. Donnelly DE, Morrison PJ. Ulster Med J. 2014 83:86-8.

Richard Kiel - obituary. The Telegraph. 11 Sep 2014.

Joseph Boruwlaski: the last court dwarf of the History. Trimarchi F. J Endocrinol Invest. 2018 41: 1357-1358.

Lionel Messi's improbable progression from struggling youngster to world super star. Balague G. The Telegraph. Dec 2 2013

The Illnesses and Death of Queen Mary I. Abernethy S. The Freelance History Writer. Feb 23, 2018

Hyperprolactinemia. Majumdar A, Mangal NS. J Hum Reprod Sci. 2013. 6: 168–175.

The Tragic True Story Behind Peter Dinklage's Latest Role. Nicolaou E. Refinery29. Oct 19 2018.

Gail Devers: 'A girl asked what was wrong with me. She said I looked like a monster' J Jackson. The Guardian. April 1 2007.

Thomas Addison's disease after 154 years: modern diagnostic perspectives on an old condition L. Leelarathna, J.K. Powrie, P.V. Carroll. QJM: An International Journal of Medicine, 2009 102, 8, 569–573.

A new view of JFK's Addison's disease. Maugh II TH. Los Angeles Times. Sep 5, 2009.

Jane Austen and Addison's disease: An unconvincing diagnosis. White C. Medical Humanities. 2009. 35:98-100.

Cushing's disease: pathobiology, diagnosis, and management. Lonser RR, Nieman L, Oldfield EH. literature review J Neurosurg 126:404–417, 2017.

Hypothesis: King Henry VIII's (1491-1547) personality change: A case of lead poisoning? Charlton A. J Med Biogr. 2017. 25(2):72-80.

Elvis Presley: Head Trauma, Autoimmunity, Pain, and Early Death. Tennant F,. Practical Pain Management. 2016. 9, 13;5

Steve Redgrave: 'I feared diabetes would end my rowing career. Johnson S. The Guardian. June 12 2018

'I inject five times a day,' Theresa May reveals as she talks openly about living with diabetes. Hope C. The Guardian. May 5 2017.

Olympic swimmer defies odds against diabetes. Carney K. CNN Headline News. Sep 5, 2003

Intersex and proud: model Hanne Gaby Odiele on finally celebrating her body. Hicklin A. The Telegraph. April 23 2017

Human Heredity: Principles and Issues. Cummings M, 2009.

5α-Reductase: History and Clinical Importance. Marks LS. Rev Urol. 2004; 6(Suppl 9): S11–S21.

Mammalian sexual differentiation: lessons from the spotted hyena. Glickman SE, Cunha GR, Drea CM, Conley AJ, Place NJ. Trends in Endocrinology and Metabolism 2006 17; 9, 349-356

Herculine Barbin: Being the Recently Discovered Memoirs of a Nineteenth-century French Hermaphrodite. Barbin, Herculine; Foucault M. 1980. New York: Pantheon Books

The woman who didn't realise she was female until she was 19. Smith M. WalesOnline. Mar 28 2018.

## METABOLIC DISORDERS

Inborn errors of metabolism and expanded newborn screening: review and update. Mak CM, Lee HC, Chan AY, Lam CW. Crit Rev Clin Lab Sci. 2013 Nov;50(6):142-62.

Newborn blood spot test. NHS. https://www.nhs.uk/conditions/pregnancy-and-baby/newborn-blood-spot-test/ retrieved July 2 2019.

Phenylketonuria. NHS. https://www.nhs.uk/conditions/phenylketonuria/

Archaeology: The milk revolution. Curry A. Nature vol 500. Aug 1 2013

Asbjørn Følling and the discovery of phenylketonuria. Christ SE. J Hist Neurosci. 2003 Mar;12(1):44-54.

Pearl S. Buck and phenylketonuria (PKU). Finger S, Christ SE. J Hist Neurosci. 2004 Mar;13(1):44-57.

How a community stamped out Tay Sachs disease with genetic screening. Henderson M. The Times. Feb 8 2010.

The severe gout of Holy Roman Emperor Charles V. Ordi J, Alonso PL, de Zulueta J, Esteban J, Velasco M, Mas E, Campo E, Fernández PL. N Engl J Med. 2006 Aug 3;355(5):516-20.

## VISUAL DISORDERS

Genotype–phenotype associations and human eye color. White D, Rabago-Smith M. Journal of Human Genetics. 2011. 56, 5–7.

Tanna P, Strauss RW, Fujinami K, et al Stargardt disease: clinical features, molecular genetics, animal models and therapeutic options British Journal of Ophthalmology 2017;101:25-30.

No Finish Line: My Life As I See It. Runyan M, Jenkins S, Schirner E. Berkley Publishing Group, 2002

Winter Olympics 2010: Blind athlete Brian McKeever set to ski into the record books. Davies GA. The Telegraph. 10 Feb 2010.

Retinitis Pigmentosa: Genes and Disease Mechanisms. Ferrari S, Di Iorio E, Barbaro V, Ponzin D, Sorrentino FS, Parmeggiani F. Curr Genomics. 2011 Jun; 12(4): 238–249.

Eyes Wide Open: Overcoming Obstacles and Recognizing Opportunities in a World that Can't See Clearly. Isaac Lidsky. TarcherPerigee. 2017.

Retinoblastoma. NHS. https://www.nhs.uk/conditions/retinoblastoma/

Obituaries in the Performing Arts, 2011. Peter Falk. . Lentz III HM. McFarland Pub.

Caroline Aherne obituary. Jeffries S. The Telegraph. July 2 2016.

Myopic artists. Polland W. Acta Ophthalmol Scand. 2004 Jun;82(3 Pt 1):325-6.

Are we ready for genetic testing for primary open-angle glaucoma? Khawaja AP, Viswanathan AC. Eye. 2018. 32, 877–883.

The blindness of John Milton. Documenta Ophthalmologica. 1995. 89, 1–2, 15–28.

The Self-Portrait Jorge Luis Borges Drew After Going Blind. Temple E. Literary Hub. 24, 2018

Blindness of Johann Sebastian Bach. Tarkkanen A. Acta Ophthalmol. 2013. 9:191-2.

The chemistry of John Dalton's color blindness. Hunt DM, Dulai KS, Bowmaker JK, Mollon JD. Science. 1995 Feb 17;267(5200):984-8.

Colour blindness. Gordon N. Public Health. 1998. 112, 2, 81-84.

The Lindbergh of Canada: The Erroll Boyd Story. Smyth R. 1997

Colorblindness Gene Found in Pacific Islanders. Brown V. Science Jun. 26, 2000.

Magic Carpet Ride: The Autobiography of John Kay and Steppenwolf. Quarry Press,Canada (Aug. 1994).

A "Fille du Roy" Introduced the T14484C Leber Hereditary Optic Neuropathy Mutation in French Canadians. Laberge AM, Jomphe M, Houde L, Vézina H, Tremblay M, Desjardins B, Labuda D, St-Hilaire M, Macmillan C, Shoubridge EA, Brais B. Am J Hum Genet. 2005 Aug; 77(2): 313–317.

Scottsdale's Scott MacIntyre: More on the American Idol Contestant. Cizmar M. Phoenix New Times. Jan 13 2009.

What was the matter with Dr Spooner? Jay B. 1987. Br Med J. 17;295:942-3.

The diagnosis of art: Durer's squint – and Shakespeare's? Aronson JK, Ramachandran M. J R Soc Med. 2009. 102:391-3.

## HEARING AND BALANCE DISORDERS

Hearing loss and connexin 26. Kemperman MH, Hoefsloot LH, Cremers CWRJ. J R Soc Med. 2002 Apr; 95(4): 171–177.

Detection of epidermal thickening in GJB2 carriers with epidermal US. Guastalla P, Guerci VI, Fabretto A, Faletra F, Grasso DL, Zocconi E, Stefanidou D, D'Adamo P, Ronfani L, Montico M, Morgutti M, Gasparini P. Radiology. 2009. 251:280-6.

The deafness of Beethoven: an audiologic and medical overview. Shearer PD.

Am J Otol. 1990 Sep;11(5):370-4.

Dina Carroll, Biography. http://dinacarroll.com/bio. Accessed July 2 2019.

Frankie Valli Biography. https://www.biography.com/musician/frankie-valli

Waardenburg syndrome. Read AP, Newton VE. J MedGenet. 1997. 34:656-665

Congenital Deafness with Cardiac Arrhythmias: The Jervell and Lange-Nielsen Syndrome. Wahl RA, Macdonald Dick II. American Annals of the Deaf. 1980. 125, 1, 34-37.

John Tracy, 82; deaf son of actor Spencer Tracy, clinic namesake. Nelson VJ. Los Angeles Times. June 17 2007.

The black paintings and the Vogt-Koyanagi-Harada syndrome. Vargas LM. J Fla Med Assoc. 1995. 82, 533-4.

The health of Jonathan Swift. Bewley TH. J R Soc Med. 1998. 91: 602-5.

Scenes from Andrew Kötting's life. Sandhu S. The Telegraph. Nov 18 2011.

## PERIPHERAL NERVOUS SYSTEM DISORDERS

Charcot-Marie-Tooth disease. NHS https://www.nhs.uk/conditions/ charcot-marie-tooth-disease/

MacCulloch: Please, don't feel sorry for me. Stein M. ESPN. 3 Mar, 2003.

Catwoman – A Superhero With Charcot-Marie-Tooth. Tresca I. CMT Journal.

Augusto Odone obituary. Stanford P. the Telegraph. Nov 1 2013.

Origin of Friedreich's disease in Quebec. Barbeau A, Sadibelouiz M, Roy M, Lemieux B, Bouchard JP, Geoffroy G. Can J Neurol Sci. 1984.11, 4 :506-9.

Philip E. B. Jourdain (1879-1919). Jourdain L. https://www.journals.uchicago.edu/doi/pdfplus/10.1086/358124

Spectrin mutations cause spinocerebellar ataxia type 5. Ikeda Y, Dick KA, Weatherspoon MR, Gincel D, Armbrust KR, Dalton JC, Stevanin G, Dürr A, Zühlke C, Bürk K, Clark HB, Brice A, Rothstein JD, Schut LJ, Day JW, Ranum LP. Nat Genet. 2006 Feb;38(2):184-90.

## CENTRAL NERVOUS SYSTEM DISORDERS

National Center for Biotechnology Information (US). Genes and Disease. Bethesda (MD): NCBI (US); 1998-. The Nervous System.

Einstein and Newton showed signs of autism. Muir H. New Scientist. April 30 2003.

Syd Barrett, Founder of Pink Floyd band, Sufferer of Schizophrenia, Passed Away this

Week." Schizophrenia Daily News Blog. 12 July 2006

The Peter Green Story - Man of the World [DVD]. Wienerworld. Oct 23 2017.

Funny Is Money. Ben Stiller and the dilemma of modern stardom. Friend T. The New Yorker. June 18, 2012.

The Darker Side of Owen Wilson. Keegan RW TIME. Aug. 29, 2007

People with learning disabilities in England 2015: Main report. https://www.gov.uk/government/publications/people-with-learning-disabilities-in-england-2015

Terry Pratchett and his rare Alzheimer's diagnosis. Shakespeare T. Alzheimers Society. Feb 11 2017.

Harold Wilson'may have had Alzheimer's when he resigned. Morris N. The Independent. Nov 11 2008.

Ronald Reagan had Alzheimer's while president, says son. Pilkington E. The Guardian. Jan 17 2011.

Dudley Moore dies at 66. Jeffery S. The Guardian. 27 Mar 2002.

Robin. Dave Itzkoff. Holt H. 2018

Did Immanuel Kant have dementia with Lewy bodies and REM behavior disorder? Miranda M, Slachevsky A, Garcia-Borreguero D. Sleep Med. 2010. 11: 586-8.

Dementia with Lewy bodies and the neurobehavioral decline of Mervyn Peake. Sahlas DJ. Arch Neurol. 2003 Jun;60(6):889-92.

Scrooge 'was a victim of brain disease'. Harlow J. The Sunday Times. Dec 24 2006.

Michael's Story. The Michael J. Fox Foundation for Parkinson's Research. Accessed June 2 2019.

Ozzy Osbourne: The Prince of Darkness sheds a little light on whether this truly is the end. Yarborough C. Cleveland.com. Sep 10 2018

Adolf Hitler and His Parkinsonism. Bhattacharyya KB. Ann Indian Acad Neurol. 2015 Oct-Dec; 18(4): 387–390.

The Cognitive Neuropsychiatry of Parkinson's Disease. Famous people suspected of having PD. McNamara P. Sentinel. 2012.

The Huntington disease of woody guthrie: another man done gone. Ringman JM. Cogn

Behav Neurol. 2007. 20: 238-43.

The story of George Huntington and his disease. Bhattacharyya KB. Ann Indian Acad Neurol. 2016. 19: 25–28.

The History of George Balanchine and the New York City Ballet. Gottlieb R. Vanity Fair Dec 1998.

The Family That Couldn't Sleep: A Medical Mystery Paperback. Max DT. Random House Trade Paperbacks. 2007.

Kuru: A Journey Back in Time from Papua New Guinea to the Neanderthals' Extinction. Liberski PP. Pathogens. 2013 Sep; 2(3): 472–505.

## GENES AND CANCER

The Genetics of Cancer Risk. Pomerantz MM, Freedman ML. Cancer J. 2011. 17:416-22.

Early History of Cancer. The American Cancer Society medical and editorial content team. Jan 4, 2018.

Death at 32 of fashion leader Reza. Bailey S. Bournmouth Daily Echo. May 23 2008.

Actress Christina Applegate reveals she had her ovaries, fallopian tubes removed. Freydkin D. TODAY. Oct. 11, 2017

Angelina Jolie effect' boosted genetic testing rates, study suggests. Davis N. The Guardian. Dec 14 2016.

Monopolizing Our Bodies? The Myriad Supreme Court Case and Issues of Access and Justice. Elster N, Parsi K. Current Obstetrics and Gynecology Reports. 2013. 2, 4, 196–198.

Did Adrenal Tumors Fuel the Hatfield-McCoy Feud? A rare disease has been found in West Virginia McCoy descendants. Psychology Today. Sarkis SA. May 29 2012.

NBA Great Kareem Abdul-Jabbar Diagnosed With Leukemia Netter S. abcNEWS. Nov. 10, 2009

## DNA REPAIR AND PREMATURE AGEING

DNA repair diseases: What do they tell us about cancer and aging? Menck CFM, Munford V. Genet Mol Biol. 2014. 37: 220–33.

PROFILE: Riley McCoy lives with Xeroderma Pigmentosum. The Orange Country Register. Nov 19, 2007

Progeria sufferer Hayley Okines dies, aged 17. Harley N. The Telegraph. Apr 3 2015.

Hutchinson-Gilford Progeria syndrome: its presentation in F. Scott Fitzgerald's short story 'The Curious Case of Benjamin Button' and its oral manifestations. Maloney WJ. J Dent Res. 2009 Oct;88(10):873-6.

## DNA: PAST, PRESENT & FUTURE

Friedrich Miescher and the discovery of DNA. Dahm R. Dev Biol. 2005 Feb 15;278(2):274-88. Review.

Oswald Avery, DNA, and the transformation of biology. Cobb M. Curr Biol. 2014 Jan 20;24(2):R55-60. Review

Francis Crick: Discoverer of the Genetic Code. Matt Ridley

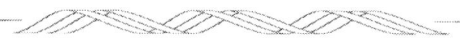

# Illustrations

Cover; C.Murgatroyd; Drawing of a Purkinje cell in the cat's cerebellar cortex, by Santiago Ramón y Cajal, adapted from an old Grey's Anatomy, source Wikipedia, Monastery cells and biological cells, Diagram of a cell, DNA replication, The Central Dogma, Translation of RNA all by C. Murgatroyd; Frederich Sanger, source www,nlm.nih.gov/visibleproofs/media/ gallery/vi_a_208b; DNA wraps around histones by C. Murgatroyd; Genetic Inheritance, anonymous; Gregor Mendel, source www,malaspina.com/jpg/mendel.jpg; Inheritance of flower colour, Inheritance of Habsburg jaw, Punnet squares, Inheritance of earlobe form, Example of inheritance, Part of possible Ptolemaic genealogy, Family tree of the British and European Royal families, The family of Tsar Nicholas II, The Julio-Claudian family tree, A male donkey crossed all by C. Murgatroyd; Boy with a puppet by Giovanni Caroto, source Wikipedia; Billy Bunter by C.H.Chapman, source Wikipedia; Audrey Hepburn, Paramount-photo by Bud Fraker; A punnet square showing inheritance of ear form, Bottleneck diagram, Founder effect diagram, Strand of DNA all by C. Murgatroyd; Chromosomes, source Wikipedia; Human chromosomes by Steffen Dietzel; A Calico cat by M.Carroll; Madelaine Stuart, Madelinemgmt; Eva Klobukowska by J.Szewiński, H. Sourek; Lili Elbe by Gerta Gottlieb source Wikipedia; Bone by M.Carroll; Peter Dinklage by Mia Tomova; The Ovitz family, source Wikipedia; Verne Troyer by Mia Tomova; Warick Davis by Mia Tomova; Ellis van Crevald syndrome by Victor McKusick; Lucia Zarate, source Wikipedia; Henri de Toulouse-Lautrec, 1894, source Paul Sescau40002; Egill Skallagrímsson, 17th century Icelandic manuscript AM 426 fol., now in the care of the Árni Magnússon Institute in Iceland; Rocky Dennis, source 1977 Jr. High school yearbook; Glendora, California; Skeleton of Harry Eastlack by Joh-co;

diseases, syphilology and dermatology (1893) by Morrow, Prince A; Bart de Graaf, by KRO-91876-kb12-8 pos.png; Intestines by M.Carroll; Eighteenth-century engraving of the early English king Eadred. National Potrait Gallery (ER14678); Blood cells by M.Carroll; Sickle cell By Gregory Kato - Own work, CC BY-SA 4.0; Miles Davis, à Antibes dans la nuit du 26 au 27 juillet 1963. À gauche, Ron Carter. À droite, Tony Williams; Pete Sampras by Craig ONeal, CC BY-SA 2.0; broad beans by Tuinboon_zaden_in_peul; Metabolic pathway for heme synthesis by C. Murgatroyd; Bela Lugosi as Count Dracula, source Wikipedia; George III by Allan Ramsey, source Wikipedia; Ero Mantytranta, source Wikipedia; Alexi Nicholaevitch Romanov, Boasson and Eggler St. Petersburg Nevsky 24; Robert Louis Stevenson, Photograph by Henry Walter Barnett, 1893, State Library of New South Wales; Immune cells from "Manual of pathology : including bacteriology, the technic of postmortems, and methods of pathologic research" (1905) by Coplin, William Michael Late; The Plague of Athens, Michiel Sweerts, c.1652–1654, Gift of The Ahmanson Foundation (AC1997.10.1); David Vetter, source Wikipedia; Seal, By Siebbi - CC BY 3.0; Endocrine System by M.Carroll; Hypothalamus and pituitary gland by M.Carroll; Charles Byrne by J. Kay., source Wikipedia; Richard Kiel by Mia Tomova; Rondo Hatton, cartuneland.com, photo of an oil painting; Józef Boruwlaski, anonymous, source Wikipedia; Lionel Messi By Agencia de Noticias; Mary I of England by Antonis Mor; Thyroid gland by M.Carroll; Herve Villechaize, source Wiipedia; Adrenal Gland by M.Carroll; Gail Devers, source 2.0 Generic (CC BY 2.0). John F Kennedy, source Wikipedia; Elvis Presley, Ollie Atkins, chief White House photographer; Sir Steve Redgrave in his first kayak race by Ollie Harding www.paddlepics.co.uk; Metabolism of testosterone by C.Murgatroyd; Hanne Gaby Odiele, By Ed Kavishe/fashionwirepress.com; Joan of Arc, anonymous, source Wikipedia; Female spotted hyena by M.Carroll; Still Life with Carafe, Bottle, and Fruit, Paul Cezanne, 1906, Henry and Rose Pearlman Collection; Ivar Asbjorn Folling, Wikipedia; Charles V of Spain by Lambert Sustris, source Wikipedia; Eye by M.Carroll; Elizabeth Taylor from the October 1954 issue of Modern Screen magazine; Kate Bosworth at the Deauville film festival by Georges Biard; Coloboma by Jmarchn; Peter Falk, source Wikipedia; the Swing by Pierre-Auguste Renoir; John Milton, Portrait

# About the author

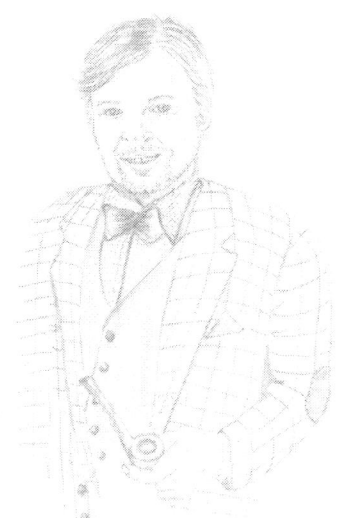

Chris Murgatroyd lectures in genetics and neuroscience at Manchester Met University. He received a Dr. rer. nat from the Ludwig Maximillians University, Munich and worked as a Postdoctoral Student at the Max-Planck Institute of Psychiatry before moving to Manchester in 2011. His major research area is in epigenetics, stress and depression. He has never owned a pipe or a jacket with elbow patches, but has always aspired to!

# Acknowledgments

Thanks go to my family and friends who have listened over the years to me talking about this book. I would like to acknowledge the students in my lectures who have listened to some of the material here and have allowed me to gauge interest. I am very much indebted to my father who has read many proofs for grammar and English and to Michael Carroll for many ideas. Thanks again to Michael and to Mia Tamova for illustrations and all the individuals who have allowed copy-right free access to photographs.

Printed in Great Britain
by Amazon